KU-162-310

PENGUIN BOOKS

LIVING WITH ALZHEIMER'S DISEASE AND SIMILAR CONDITIONS

Doctor Gordon Wilcock is Professor and Head of the Department of Care of the Elderly at Bristol University and a Consultant at Frenchay Hospital in Bristol. He is one of the founders of the Alzheimer's Disease Society, of which he was the Chairman from 1979 to 1986, and is currently a Vice President and serves on the Society's Medical Panel, of which he was formerly Chairman. He is also involved in research into Alzheimer's disease and similar conditions. His books include *Our Elders* and *Pocket Consultant in Geriatrics*, and he is a co-editor of an international, multidisciplinary manual providing advice for doctors and other professionals caring for people with dementia. In addition, he has had numerous articles published in medical journals.

DR GORDON WILCOCK

Living with Alzheimer's Disease

and similar conditions

A Guide for Families and Carers

New Edition

PENGUIN BOOKS

PENGUIN BOOKS

Published by the Penguin Group
Penguin Books Ltd, 27 Wrights Lane, London w8 5tz, England
Penguin Putnam Inc., 375 Hudson Street, New York, New York 10014, USA
Penguin Books Australia Ltd, Ringwood, Victoria, Australia
Penguin Books Canada Ltd, 10 Alcorn Avenue, Toronto, Ontario, Canada m4v 3b2
Penguin Books (NZ) Ltd, Private Bag 102902, NSMC, Auckland, New Zealand

Penguin Books Ltd, Registered Offices: Harmondsworth, Middlesex, England

First published 1990
This edition published 1999
10 9 8 7 6 5 4 3 2 1

Set in 11/13pt Monotype Ehrhardt
Typeset by Rowland Phototypesetting Ltd, Bury St Edmunds, Suffolk
Printed in England by Clays Ltd, St Ives plc

Contents

Acknowledgements

The author would like to thank all those who have taught him so much during the last twenty years or so about the problems of caring for a loved one with dementia, and how they have helped themselves and others to cope. These people who have given generously of their advice have included families of carers, members of the Alzheimer's Disease Society and sometimes even sufferers themselves. It is to them that this book is especially dedicated. Finally I would like to thank my family for gracefully accepting my prolonged absences at weekends whilst writing.

Preface

Much has happened since I wrote the first edition of this book. Research has marched on in leaps and bounds and much of our new knowledge has been included in the relevant chapters, particularly where it relates to a better understanding of what is happening in the brain in people with dementia, and in relation to the development of treatment strategies, including the drugs that are now available to help with the symptoms.

Our new knowledge is also important in relation to our understanding of how changes in the blood supply to the brain can produce dementia. In addition, a new type of dementia has begun to emerge as an entity in its own right, dementia associated with Lewy bodies.

This new information has necessitated much re-writing of some of the chapters, and also the creation of a new chapter about Lewy body dementia. Nevertheless, the basic structure of the book is unchanged, with the first section devoted to background knowledge and understanding of what is happening within the brain and also the benefits of research. The second section contains what I hope will be helpful advice, most contributed by carers over the years, to whom I am very grateful.

As in the first edition, the most important message that this book is intended to deliver is that of hope and encouragement. The development of dementia in a person you love is indeed a devastating experience and the way forward can be long and difficult. Nevertheless, much can be done to maintain and improve the quality of life of both the person with dementia and those who care for and about them. The main purpose of this book is to maximize the positive side to caring.

Finally, I do hope that any readers who feel they have a contribution that might be usefully considered for the next edition, should there be one, will write to me. All suggestions will be seriously considered and the feedback gratefully received.

Gordon Wilcock
July 1998

Introduction

Alzheimer's disease is an illness that will affect the lives of many of us, directly or indirectly, in the coming years, and this book has been written to provide support, guidance and information on the subject. It is intended mainly for relatives who find themselves having to look after someone who is suffering from a dementing illness, but it also contains much information that should be of assistance to professional carers and those working with voluntary organizations. It should help people make the most of the resources available and improve as much as possible the quality of life of a person suffering from Alzheimer's disease or a similar disorder.

The background to Alzheimer's disease and other illnesses that cause dementia forms the subject of some of the earlier chapters. Much of our hope for the future is invested in the enormous amount of research that is being undertaken all over the world to help develop new and more effective approaches to treatment and ultimately to identify the causes, so that one day we may be in a position to prevent people contracting this terrible illness. Some of the more important research is described in later chapters, especially chapter 7. Since the first edition of this book, research has made important strides and not only do we now have a much greater understanding and knowledge of the abnormal processes that Alzheimer's disease and other dementias cause in the brain, but we now have some treatments that improve the quality of life of a significant proportion of people with Alzheimer's disease. Although this is only the beginning, as far as drug treatment is concerned, it is a major step forward and further, and hopefully more effective, treatments are in the pipeline.

The greater part of the book explains the ways in which a person's illness affects him or her and also those who are in a caring role. There is practical advice on how to cope with the physical and psychological problems that occur in those suffering from a dementing illness, and also advice for carers about the problems that may well affect them too.

In addition to being involved in treating people with dementia in my day-to-day work and offering advice to carers, I have been privileged to gain a much wider insight into the problems from my experience in the voluntary sector – particularly the Alzheimer's Disease Society, which I helped to found in 1979. Much of what is written in this book is based upon discussions I have had with sufferers and those caring for them. It also draws upon the advice that has been given by countless relatives, friends and professional carers on coping with the problems they have encountered.

What is dementia?

Dementia is caused by many different illnesses that can affect the brain, and a lot of confusing terminology has arisen. This can lead to misunderstanding, not only in the minds of lay people but also among the medical and associated professions. The term dementia means simply a reduction in or impairment of mental powers. It does not mean that a person is mad – indeed often the only early sign is an exaggeration of the memory loss that so many of us suffer as we grow older, though most people who are forgetful are not suffering from, and will never develop, dementia. As is explained later, dementia eventually involves far more than memory loss; symptoms may include disorientation in time, a tendency to become lost in familiar surroundings, difficulty in recognizing objects or people, and eventually an inability to carry out previously familiar tasks. The fact that several mental abilities are affected is one of the hallmarks of dementia although of course, to begin with, the impairment of mental functioning is less.

It is important also to realize what is not dementia. Dementia is very definitely not a part of normal ageing, and can in fact occur in quite young people, although not as frequently as in those who are over the age of seventy-five. It is also not a diagnosis. The term dementia merely describes the state that a person's mind is in, the way it is working or not working, a person's behaviour pattern, and so on. It is rather akin to saying that one is short of breath. In the case of breathlessness something has usually affected the way in which the lungs or the heart work, and it is the underlying cause of this, for example pneumonia or a heart attack, that is the true diagnosis.

Many conditions cause dementia. The most common is Alzheimer's disease and although it can occur in people who are old or young, it very rarely occurs before the age of forty-five. The next most common cause of dementia is probably a disturbance of the blood supply to the brain. This can occur as a series of small strokes, which cause the death of brain cells, and which may show none of the usual manifestations of a stroke, i.e. there is no evidence of a paralysed arm or leg. We used to think that multiple small strokes were the main cause of vascular dementia but we now know that there are many other changes that can affect the blood supply to the brain and result in a dementia. Evidence is now emerging that even Alzheimer's disease itself may have a vascular component, but at the time of writing this has not definitely been proved.

The third common cause of dementia is known as 'Lewy body dementia', because the affected brain cells contain an abnormal structure, the Lewy body, named after the doctor who first described them. Although this is not the same type of dementia as that which sometimes occurs in patients with Parkinson's disease who develop dementia, there is some overlap with this condition. Some doctors believe that Lewy body dementia is the second commonest cause and occurs more frequently than vascular dementia. At the moment this is a matter of debate but it does not really matter very much. What is important is to remember that there are three common causes of dementia – Alzheimer's disease, vascular dementia and dementia associated with Lewy bodies.

Alzheimer's disease is named after the German doctor Alois Alzheimer who first described it in detail in 1907. The changes in the brain, described in more detail in later chapters, are caused by a slowly progressive loss of the nerve cells lying in the *cerebral cortex* – the thin rim of grey matter on the outside of the brain – and in other collections of nerve cells lying more deeply within the brain. Alzheimer's disease is the commonest cause of dementia and on its own, or in combination with one of the other conditions, contributes to the dementia in between 50 and 70 per cent of patients who develop such a condition. Many different causes probably contribute to its development and most doctors now realize that it is probably not a simple single condition, but multifactorial in its origins.

There are of course many other causes of dementia; some of them, albeit a minority, are curable, which is why it is so important that a proper diagnosis of the underlying illness is always made. These causes will be described in later chapters.

Many other terms for describing the condition are in common use, among them *chronic brain failure*, *organic brain failure*, *organic brain syndrome*, *hardening of the arteries*, and *senility*. The latter is an unfortunate term and implies that the condition is associated with ageing, which in turn implies that it is inevitable and untreatable. All of these alternative terms should be avoided as they are a 'hangover' from old concepts that are now largely abandoned and have been replaced by the use of the term dementia as a description of what has happened to the sufferer, followed by the need to make a diagnosis of which illness is causing the dementia, i.e. is Alzheimer's disease or another condition responsible?

It is essential to realize that dementia is not the same as the more short-term episodes of confusion that are suffered by many old people as a result of infections such as pneumonia or urinary tract infection, the side-effects of drugs, or as a consequence of other medical conditions. These are more correctly called *acute confusional states* and don't produce the gradual and relentlessly progressive deterioration in mental functioning that is a feature of dementia; on the contrary, the onset is usually fairly rapid and the sufferer is often in a state of semi-consciousnes or sub-consciousness. The most common example of this is the delirium associated with a high fever.

Finally, there is a lot of misunderstanding about the role of 'hardening of the arteries' or *arteriosclerosis*. These two terms essentially mean the same thing, and are often used to describe the condition that is causing a person's dementia. This dates back to an extremely old-fashioned and incorrect belief that hardening of the arteries narrowed them to such an extent that the whole brain, or parts of it, had its blood supply slowly strangled and in consequence could not work properly. It has been known since the early seventies that this is not the case, yet it is still given as the diagnosis by many doctors.

The size of the problem

Dementia probably afflicts in the region of a half to three-quarters of a million people in the UK. It is therefore a problem that surpasses AIDS in its magnitude and, unlike AIDS, many of the causes of dementia, especially Alzheimer's disease, are conditions for which there are no known preventative measures currently available. It is often estimated that approximately 7 to 10 per cent of the population aged sixty-five and over suffer from one of the dementias. *This of course means that most people are not so afflicted and are, therefore, in a position to help those less fortunate than themselves.* Clearly, those suffering from dementia are unable to improve their lot on their own, and cannot lobby for better facilities and care for themselves, or greater support for those looking after them. It is a great scandal that even in such a civilized society as ours, it is those who can make the biggest noise about their plight, or who command a significant proportion of the vote, that are most likely to advance their position.

The size of the problem is going to escalate rapidly, especially in the next twenty years. Although less than one person in one thousand under the age of sixty-five years suffers with a dementia, the situation changes as the years advance. Of those aged sixty-five to seventy, it appears that approximately one person in twenty has dementia, but the proportion of sufferers rises with increasing age, and of those over the age of seventy-five, one person in five will probably have some degree of dementia. The number of older people in our population is expected to increase greatly between now and the early years of the next century, and by far the largest proportional increase will be in those aged seventy-five and over. This means, of course, that the growing number of elderly people suffering with dementia is going to make greater and greater demands upon the rest of society, unless effective treatment or preventative measures become available in the near future.

In approximately 10 per cent of people suffering from dementia up to the age of sixty-five, the underlying cause will be remediable. In older people, especially those over the age of seventy, this figure probably falls to 5 per cent, one person in twenty. This is nevertheless a significant and important number of people for whom treatment can alleviate an otherwise bleak future. Treatment of some of the underlying conditions will not necessarily reverse the dementia and may only stop it from getting worse, but everybody who develops dementia should be screened for the underlying illness that is causing it as early as possible to limit the damage that is done before treatment is started. The treatments mentioned in this paragraph refer to conditions such as vitamin deficiencies, glandular abnormalities and so on. The early treatments now available for Alzheimer's disease are moving it into the 'treatable' category, but these new treatments in reality probably only help with symptoms, whilst correcting a vitamin deficiency or a glandular disorder in those who have one is, of course, remedying the underlying illness completely. I hope it will not be many years before we will have a similar approach to the treatment of Alzheimer's disease, but at the moment we are limited to reducing the impact of the disease processes on a patient's symptoms, and are not yet able to cure the underlying disease mechanism itself.

Even in those in whom the dementia proves to be untreatable, once a diagnosis has been made it is easier to plan the future, advise relatives or other carers of what the future may hold and how they can best prepare themselves for what lies ahead. A lot of support is usually available, far more than is often realized, and access to this is facilitated once the diagnosis is known and accepted. In those parts of the country where sadly there is little or no support, knowledge of the diagnosis may allow relatives to get together to try and help each other and to lobby for more resources.

Summary

When a diagnosis of 'dementia' is made, it is essential not to accept this on its own but to insist that a proper diagnosis of the underlying cause is made, as early in the course of the illness as possible, in case the underlying cause is treatable. The family, or others who are in a caring role, can then make sure that they are aware of what is available locally by way of support from both the statutory bodies – the health service and social services – and also from the voluntary sector, such as the Alzheimer's Disease Society. Where the provision of support is inadequate, if a group of carers gets together they may be able to press for better resources more effectively than individuals on their own.

If someone you care about has an illness causing dementia the path ahead may be a long and difficult one, but advice and support is becoming increasingly available. The purpose of this book is to try to help lighten your load, while at the same time assisting you to improve the quality of life of the person who is afflicted.

I

The Normal Brain and How It Ages

Our brain is such an important part of our body, even of our very existence, that it is protected within the skull by the bones of the cranial cavity. Any damage to the head sufficient to break the skull bones has serious consequences for the brain, ranging from loss of consciousness to permanent brain damage, with subsequent impairment of intellect or of physical body function.

It is less well known that the brain also has other protective systems. These consist of a series of membranes and a fluid known as the *cerebro-spinal fluid* (CSF). These are arranged in such a way that the brain is enclosed within a tough outer membrane, or sac, called the *dura mater*, and within this lies another sac containing the CSF and the brain. Suspending the brain within the bag of fluid protects it not only from the day-to-day jolts that it would otherwise receive, but also from more serious damage – say a blow on the head that is insufficient to fracture the skull bones. Despite this protection, excessive physical force is still capable of causing damage, although this would be much greater if the fluid wasn't present. The membranes also stretch tightly between the major subdivisions of the brain, thus limiting the degree to which any part of the brain can be displaced if physical trauma occurs. Our brain is therefore very well protected from the outside world.

The brain is a pinkish structure, the pink colour coming from the blood that is circulating in the minute blood vessels that nourish the nerve cells. Each brain contains some 10 to 12 billion (UK) nerve cells – also called *neurones*. The brain is so important that it takes up about 20 per cent of the blood that our hearts pump out, and consumes a similar amount of the oxygen that we breathe in through our lungs. Despite requiring such a large amount of blood and oxygen it weighs only a fraction of our total body weight, usually in the region of 2–3lb (1–1.5kg).

It is often assumed that the larger a person's brain the more intelligent they are; this is fine for male chauvinists as in general men appear to have larger brains than women! Sadly, however, at least for us men, intelligence or other aspects of mental ability are not related to the size of the brain.

In order to allow us to understand more easily some of the illnesses that cause dementia, this chapter will describe some aspects of the structure of the brain, and how it works. The brain is, however, such an enormously complex organ that it would be confusing, and to a certain extent irrelevant, to explore these subjects at other than a simple level. The description that follows is, therefore, particularly arranged to take into account structures and functions that are important for the understanding of some of the dementing conditions.

The structure of the brain

The brain can be divided in simple terms into four parts. Two of these are the *cerebral hemispheres*, a left and a right, stretching from just behind the eye to the back of the head. Each hemisphere is divided into four different *lobes*. The lobe at the front – that which is just behind the eye – is called the *frontal lobe*, and amongst its many functions is the control of our behavioural pattern.

Behind the frontal lobe is the *parietal lobe* and behind that, at the back, is the *occipital lobe*. The parietal lobe has many functions and is probably best considered as one of the most important parts of the brain for the interpretation and correlation of sensory input – what we can feel when we touch something or are touched. It is also responsible for our interpretation of our body image, that is, our image of our own bodies. Damage to this system may result in an individual neglecting a useful limb or failing to recognize that a limb is paralysed, as occurs after some strokes. It is also responsible for coordinating some functional activities, so that damage to it may result in an inability to execute planned movements, for example doing up buttons. This should be distinguished from a similar difficulty that can result from damage to nerves and muscles. The occipital lobe is important for the interpretation of visual sensation and damage to it will result in disturbance of vision.

The fourth lobe of the brain, the *temporal lobe*, which lies a little below the parietal lobe and behind that part of the skull that is often referred to as our 'temple', is important for many of the dementias, especially Alzheimer's disease. In lower forms of animal life it is particularly concerned with taste and smell, as it is also in humans. In us, however, it is most important for the organization and processing of memory and has close connections with other areas of the brain. Loss of memory is of course one of the first early signs in the development of many dementing illnesses. The temporal lobe is also important for some aspects of hearing and speech.

As well as connections occurring within the brain between one part and another, each of the hemispheres sends out nerve fibres to the rest of the body, mainly to control what the muscles in the limbs do. They also receive fibres from sensory organs, such as those that are hidden in the skin that tell us about sensations of touch, pain and temperature. Strangely – and nobody really understands why – each hemisphere makes its connections with the other side of the body; in other words the left hemisphere controls movements in, and receives information from, the right side of the body and vice versa.

At the back of the brain, sitting below the hemispheres, is the third part, a small structure about the size of a man's thumb.

This is called the *brain-stem* and it joins the hemispheres to the spinal cord. As well as being a structure that has fibres passing through it, to and from the hemispheres and the body, it also has its own specialized functions. These include many of the nerve cells that control the muscles of our face, the muscles that move our eyes and those that are responsible for eating and swallowing, etc. It is also to this area of the brain that sensation from the face is first sent. In addition, the brain-stem contains special centres that are responsible for controlling our breathing, our heartbeat and other body functions automatically. These are, of course, vital centres that help to keep us alive and as they and many other structures are crammed together in a very small area of brain tissue, damage in the brain-stem can have a very profound effect upon the integrity of the rest of the body. The brain-stem is affected in many of the illnesses that cause dementia, but probably to a lesser extent than the cerebral hemispheres.

Sitting beneath the occipital lobes and behind the brain-stem is the fourth part, the *cerebellum*, whose importance lies in the control of the reflexes that determine our posture and the state of contraction of the muscles. It is essential for maintaining the body's equilibrium and for the performance of smoothly coordinated muscular actions. It is involved in some types of dementia, but not very much, if at all, in the commoner illnesses that cause intellectual impairment.

Within the brain are hollow spaces that contain the same fluid, the CSF, that has been mentioned already. The CSF in these hollow spaces, which are called *ventricles*, escapes through small openings to join the CSF that is contained within the membranes surrounding the brain. A disturbance to this system can result in a particular form of dementia that will be described in a later chapter.

The brain is, roughly speaking, also divided up into *white matter* and *grey matter*. The grey matter is not really grey in the living brain but is so described because of the appearance it takes on when it is treated in a laboratory in a particular way after a person has died. It is these grey areas that contain the bodies of the nerve cells, as described below. The largest collection of grey matter lies on the outside of our brains, rather like the rind of an orange, and it is called the *cerebral cortex*. This structure is affected in many of the dementing illnesses. Buried deep within the brain are other collections of grey matter, some of which are also affected in some of the conditions that cause dementia.

The white matter is only white because it contains a lot of fatty material. This is made up of nerve fibres which pass from the cell bodies to other areas of the brain or the body – the arms and legs for example. Most of these nerve fibres are surrounded by a fatty material which has an important function in helping messages travel down the fibres. It is this fatty material that is white, giving the brain its characteristic appearance. In summary, therefore, the brain can be considered to contain grey matter, made up of the cell bodies (the cell body is the power house of a nerve cell), and white matter, which consists of the fibres either connecting different nerve cells, or parts of them, or travelling to the rest of the body outside the brain.

Brain cells

The most important cells in the brain, the neurones which make up the grey matter, consist of a cell body and the nerve fibres passing from it. The cell body, as already mentioned, is the powerhouse of the neurone and contains a structure called the *nucleus*, from which emanate nearly all the instructions for the biochemical processes that occur within the rest of the cell. There is one major nerve fibre called the *axon* and this can be very long. The end of the axon usually breaks up into many branches, each of which makes contact with the cell body or branches of nerve fibres from other cells. Those that leave the brain either make contact with other nerve cells, in the spinal cord for example, or with other structures such as sensory organs or muscles. There are also numerous shorter nerve fibres attached to each cell body, and these are called *dendrites*. These make contact with parts of many other neurones. It is thought that some nerve cells die as people grow older, but that the branching of the remaining nerve fibres increases to make up the connections that are lost because some cells have died. It seems as if in some types of dementia this compensatory increase in the branching is abnormal or reduced.

As well as neurones there are many other types of cell in the brain. These are usually described collectively as *neuroglia*. There are several different types of neuroglia, and the function of some of them is uncertain. It used to be considered that they had a principally supportive function but we now know about some of their other functions too. As far as the dementias are concerned, it is possible that one of the more important things neuroglia do is to produce chemicals that other brain cells need, and that this process may become disturbed, leading to a malfunction of neurones which results in their death or prevents them from working properly.

Inside each neurone lies a complicated structure of little *fibrils* and *tubules*. This is sometimes referred to as the skeleton of the cell but it is also important in the passage of substances from one end of a nerve fibre to the other. In some types of dementia, including that caused by Alzheimer's disease, it may well be that a disturbance of these structures and their transport function affects the way the nerve cells work.

The brain's message system

As has been mentioned already, nerve fibres connect with parts of other nerve cells. The message travels down the nerve fibre using a process that is often likened to an electrical current flowing down a wire. This is a convenient way of thinking about it and, although it isn't quite right, for our purposes it is a useful analogy. When it gets to the end of the nerve fibre the message has to 'switch on' the next nerve cell or one of its dendrites, and there is a special system to make this possible.

Although it looks as if the connecting parts of two nerve cells are actually in contact with each other when they are viewed through an ordinary microscope, we know from the electron microscope, which can produce an even higher magnification, that there is in fact a gap between the axon that is bringing the message and that part of the cell that is going to receive it. This gap is extremely narrow and the way the first nerve cell activates the second is by releasing a special chemical into this gap. The chemical travels across the gap until it hits a specialized area on the cell which is receiving the message, and the interaction between the chemical and the receiving area, which is called a *receptor*, switches on the second cell. This neurone then either transmits the message to further cells by a similar process, or reacts to the messages received in some other way.

These chemical messengers are known as *neurotransmitters*, and if they were to stay in the gap, which is in fact called a *synapse*, they would continue to stimulate the second nerve cell, which in many cases would result in its death as it would be over-stimulated. The body has, therefore, very cleverly arranged for other chemicals to be present at many of these synapses so that they can break down the neurotransmitter after it has done its job. In many of the illnesses that cause dementia, such as Alzheimer's disease, there is a gross disturbance of the chemical neurotransmitter system. Developing medicines to try to put this right is one of the approaches to treatment that is now showing some signs of success, as is described in a later chapter.

Physical and mental ageing

In general, as a person gets older, it would appear that his or her brain becomes smaller. It used to be thought that there was a considerable degree of wasting of brain material, or *atrophy* as it is technically called, between the ages of about twenty and seventy. This was based upon a comparison of brain weights in older people and younger people, measured at approximately the same time, for example during a study that recorded the weights of brains obtained at post-mortem examination in people who had died during, say, a two-year period. Unfortunately, this is very misleading as we know that the improvement in nutrition and general health, amongst other factors, that has occurred over the last fifty or sixty years has led to people being on average taller than their predecessors earlier this century. We also know that taller people have heavier brains. In other words, the weight of the brain in a person aged twenty in the late 1980s may be greater than the weight of a twenty-year-old's brain in 1930 because of better nutrition, etc.

The only accurate method of determining whether or not the brain does decrease in size with increasing age, and if so by how much, would be to study the same individual over a number of years, and this clearly is very difficult to do. There are, however, other indirect ways of trying to establish whether there is a true loss of weight of the brain with increasing age and it does in fact appear as if there is some atrophy, but probably not as much as was originally thought. Whether this atrophy, resulting from the loss of nerve cells and fibres, really matters is debatable. Many elderly people with apparently quite small brains, which have been assumed to have atrophied, are known to have had perfectly normal intellectual function, even if the examination has been made when they are in their nineties.

There undoubtedly are abnormalities in brain function in people as they grow older. The extent of these has, however, been exaggerated by earlier studies in which college students have been compared with older people in the community. Studies of this nature contain many sources of inaccuracy, and again the only way to obtain a true assessment of what happens to intellectual function as an individual grows older is to study the brain psychology over a number of years in each of a large number of individuals. Studies of this nature have been undertaken, and several are still underway.

As people grow older it does seem as if there is an impaired ability to retain new memories, whereas the facility for recalling long-term memory is relatively unimpaired. In addition they may be unable to recall details like a person's name, but can describe all sorts of other things about him or her, indicating that they have remembered quite a lot of relevant information. Later on, what was forgotten is often suddenly, and sometimes unexpectedly, recalled. To a lesser extent this appears to happen to many normal, younger people. It is certainly not the same as dementia, and whether it is of any real significance is uncertain. Older people also tend to become more rigid and inflexible and more conservative in their attitude to life.

In summary, our brains are complex organs that are well-protected by the bones and membranes of the skull. As we age, there are changes in brain structure and function, but these ageing changes alone do not cause dementia.

2

Understanding Dementia

As described earlier, dementia involves a progressive decline of intellectual ability. A declining memory alone is inadequate evidence upon which to make the diagnosis. In addition to the difficulty with remembering things, there is usually a progressive loss of the ability to think and to reason that can also affect other areas of mental functioning, for example emotion and behaviour. Most people, even the very old, do not become demented.

The simplest of the medical definitions of dementia is 'a global loss of intellectual function that is usually progressive, and in the majority but not all cases, irreversible'. The most important word in this definition is the use of the term 'global', as this reinforces the fact that memory loss alone is not the same as dementia, and that there have to be other aspects of abnormal mental functioning.

It has already been mentioned that hardening of the arteries by itself does not cause dementia, but there are also other misconceptions that need to be corrected. Dementia is not caused by under-use or over-use of the brain, and it affects people in all walks of life. With the exception of one or two very rare conditions it is not infectious – one person cannot transmit it to another. It is also not an inevitable consequence of ageing. Although it may sometimes appear to be precipitated by a stressful event, the most common example of this being the family who attribute the onset of dementia in one ageing parent to the strain of the bereavement and grief reaction caused by the death of the other, this is not usually so. In these circumstances careful inquiry will usually reveal that the intellectual changes had probably been present for some time before the bereavement occurred, but that the person who died was assisting the sufferer so that their waning mental abilities were less noticeable. When the spouse dies, the surviving partner is suddenly left exposed to the world at large, and his or her failings become more obvious.

There are so many different underlying conditions that can cause dementia that it is difficult to provide an overall picture of the way in which dementia affects personality and behaviour. For some of the most common causes of dementia the details are described in the appropriate chapters, but they will be seen to be very similar to the account which follows, representing a rather general picture of the features that are most frequently found in most people suffering from a dementing illness. It is very unlikely that any one person with dementia will show all the changes in behaviour described.

In the early stages, often the first thing that is noticed is that the normal degree of forgetfulness that some older people experience becomes much worse, perhaps sufficient to interfere with their day-to-day life. They may also have difficulty in understanding new information, which may have to be repeated to them several times. In many cases a person who has been house-proud is not so careful as he or she once was, and one can notice a deterioration in the cleanliness of their home, and sometimes of their clothes.

Meanwhile the forgetfulness may continue to get worse but it becomes more apparent that the major difficulty is with recent or short-term memories whereas those dating back many years, even to childhood, are preserved, sometimes in amazing detail. People with dementia may therefore forget what they had for lunch, or even that they had lunch only an hour or two ago, but recall with some precision the contents of a meal eaten on a special occasion such as a birthday sixty or more years ago. At a practical level this memory loss can be quite a problem, as it may result in kettles and saucepans being put on the cooker and allowed to boil dry, a gas stove or fire being turned on but not lit, and so on. Times become muddled and it is easy for a person with dementia to become lost in familiar places, for example when out shopping. Sometimes thoughtful relatives provide an electric cooker to replace one that runs on gas, or an electric fire to replace a gas fire in the hope of reducing the risk of fire or explosion. Unfortunately, this doesn't always help, as the person for whom it is intended may be unable to master the techniques involved in working the new apparatus, simple though they may appear to be.

Disorientation in time may lead to the person with dementia getting up in the middle of the night to go off to work to a job retired from twenty years earlier, and to which he or she would normally have set off at, say, 8.30 in the morning. On one occasion, the retired owner of a factory in his late seventies insisted on returning to his previous office at 3 a.m. each night, seven days a week. Rather than upset him, his family went along with his wishes until he insisted that other members of the staff were also there at that time. Eventually they sought medical advice and he was treated for his abnormal behaviour, so that he was once again able to sleep through the night.

These changes in behaviour may also affect the personality of sufferers and it is this that is often so hurtful and upsetting to those closest to them. Repetitive questioning, either as an expression of the need for reassurance or because the previous answer has been forgotten, constant wandering, aggression, noisiness and emotional instability take their toll, especially of those who love them.

At a variable point in the progress of the dementia, usually in the early or middle stages, language becomes affected. To begin with it may be forgetfulness of the correct word and this can often be circumvented, e.g. by asking if someone will pass the 'thing that you write with', rather than using the term 'pencil'. Sadly, however, even this ability declines. Some people with dementia become unable to understand the meanings of some words, even if they are in common everyday use, such as knife, fork or cup. If this happens early in the course of the disease it often results in frustration and irritability. Most of us from time to time forget someone's name. Nevertheless when we meet them, we know exactly who they are and can place them in the appropriate context – we remember perfectly well where we last saw them, what their job is, where they live, and so on. Often their name comes back to us out of the blue some time afterwards. This can also happen in people with dementia, to a greater extent than in the rest of us. More serious, however, is an apparently similar situation in which they forget who somebody is, not just what their name is. It can be extremely hurtful to a wife to be mistaken for her husband's former secretary and treated as such, or for a daughter to be mistaken for the sufferer's mother.

As the disease progresses, general abilities required for normal everyday life deteriorate progressively. With many of the dementing illnesses it almost appears a matter of 'last in first out': the more complex activities one learns in childhood are lost in the reverse order to that in which they were learned. Eventually sufferers may appear to lose all concern for social convention, relieving themselves in public, undressing at inappropriate times and inappropriate places, stealing, and engaging in other embarrassing forms of behaviour. Physical dependence becomes in the end considerable and even walking becomes difficult or impossible. Some but by no means all people with dementia become bedridden.

The three stages

The pattern of the symptoms and physical changes in most of the illnesses that cause dementia allows one to divide the progress of the disease into roughly three phases. These are by no means exact and they vary from individual to individual with the same condition, and from disease to disease. Nevertheless they give us a useful rule of thumb and allow us to decide whether a person with dementia is in the early, mid, or late stages of the disease. Each of these phases has a particular message and often these messages are not appreciated by those working in the medical and paramedical professions and the social services.

In the earliest phase of a dementing illness it is essential to ensure that the sufferer is properly investigated for treatable underlying conditions, as already emphasized, having first ascertained that the problems are really caused by dementia and not just a worse than average memory loss. It is this phase that is often incorrectly accepted by many relatives, friends and others as normal ageing and what one expects of somebody in their late seventies or early eighties. At this stage the dementia is usually causing significant memory loss, perhaps some disorientation in time, and a tendency to get lost in familiar places. Sufferers may become irritable as a result of their forgetfulness. Misplaced objects are often considered to have been stolen by others and some difficulty with language may occur.

It is in this early phase of dementia that depression is sometimes a major problem. Sometimes this is the result of the sufferer becoming aware of their loss of intellect and what this may mean, as well as the embarrassment caused by their symptoms, for instance the loss of memory when they are with other people. In some people, however, depression can itself produce a condition that is rather like a dementia, although it is important to appreciate that the relationship between the apparent dementia and depression requires careful unravelling. To this end it is often necessary for a doctor to prescribe a course of one of the newer antidepressants for a patient who appears to be both depressed and demented. Removing the depressive element will make clearer whether or not there really is also a dementing illness affecting that person. The newer antidepressants are usually preferable to the older type, as the former can aggravate a memory problem, have more troublesome side effects and may take longer to produce a meaningful benefit.

The next or middle phase is marked by a deterioration in ability that makes it clear to everybody that something is wrong and that it is no longer a question, even stretching the imagination considerably, that normal ageing is still the problem. This is when significant difficulty in day-to-day living presents itself. In this stage of the disease people with dementia may be completely unable to cook for themselves, shop, clean the house, or generally look after themselves. Speech becomes even more difficult, and wandering and similar behavioural abnormalities a major problem. This is a stage at which in many cases it becomes apparent to relatives that the individual concerned no longer has the personality they loved, though that person is nevertheless present in a physical sense. This can induce a sense of 'living bereavement' which may take years to come to terms with.

In the majority of medical conditions one expects the need for support and involvement of professional people to be greatest towards the end of the disease. It is not so with many of the conditions that cause dementia. It is now, in the middle stages of the disease, that the carers need the greatest amount of support, as it is at this stage that they have the most difficult problems to contend with, both those presented by the sufferer and also those that they themselves begin to experience on an emotional and personal level. These are addressed in later chapters. It is particularly important for doctors especially to be aware of this variation on the normal disease pattern.

The third and final phase that occurs in many cases is one of total dependence, sometimes associated with almost complete inactivity, whether the person who is suffering from dementia is confined to his or her bed or a combination of bed and chair. In many ways this period is met with some feeling of relief by carers. There is no longer the risk of an explosion or a fire from an incorrectly used gas stove, nor the possibility of an accident caused by a tendency to wander out into the road or by falling down stairs. The physical side of the illness becomes more apparent and it is easier for most people to relate to this. In many instances they have looked after a physically dependent person, such as a young child, in the past and caring for a person with dementia in this final phase is in many ways similar to looking after a child. The sad thing of course is that in the case of a child one anticipates that the problem will diminish as the child grows older, whilst in the case of someone with dementia it is going to get worse.

This account is probably one of the gloomier parts of this book. It has, however, been written for very positive reasons. Uncertainty about the future is one of the major problems with which those caring for people with dementia have to contend. Many of those involved in a professional capacity in providing advice and support are loath to explain about the future, often because they themselves find it too difficult to give relatives and other carers a full picture of what lies ahead of them. However, with the increasing acceptance of psychiatric illness as a physical problem like the malfunction of any other organ in the body, disorders of the brain, particularly the dementias, are increasingly discussed in the popular media and in casual conversation. Piece-meal and anecdotal accounts are often more frightening than having the matter carefully explained in the context of the help and support available. It is impossible to come to terms with and plan for the future if one doesn't know what the future holds. Unhappy though the picture is, it will be seen as the reader progresses that there is an enormous amount of support available, and also a lot that an individual carer can do to help him or herself to cope with the stresses and strains that will arise, and at the same time to help the person suffering from dementia to have as pleasant and full a life as is possible.

Many people caring for someone suffering from dementia want to know how long the disease will take to run its course. This is a difficult question to answer and it is almost impossible to fix a definite span to each of the three stages described. In most cases, however, the disease processes will run their course over a period of about five to seven years, but in some cases it may last for as long as fifteen years or more. Since it is often not appreciated that elderly people have a dementing illness when the disease is in its earliest stages, they may already be one or two years into the progression of their illness before the diagnosis is made. This means of course that the disease will appear to last for a shorter period.

In younger people, especially those under sixty, the disease often runs a more rapid course and may be two or three years less in duration. Even so, the disease may appear to last longer as it is often less likely that in younger people the early stages will be mistaken for anything other than something abnormal, whereas if the same symptoms had become apparent twenty years later, they might well have been mistaken for the changes of normal ageing.

Who is affected by dementia?

Like so many other conditions that mainly affect older people, there always seem to be more elderly women who are affected by these illnesses than men. This is probably a reflection of the fact that in general women live longer than men, the average woman of sixty-five having a reasonable chance of living into her early eighties, whereas most men of this age have a life expectancy of approximately thirteen years – into their late seventies. The situation isn't quite as simple as this, however, because there is a suggestion that women with Alzheimer's disease, the most common cause of dementia, tend to live longer than men with Alzheimer's disease. There is no obvious reason for this, but it may be that female demented patients are fitter than the men. Some of this difference in life expectancy may be a result of the earlier habits of the men who are now old, since men used to drink and smoke far more than women. It will be interesting to see whether contemporary changes in these habits will even out the difference in the length of life expected by normal old men and women, and those with a dementing illness.

There is no unequivocal evidence that dementia strikes any particular social class or professional group more than others. Certain types of illness that cause dementia occur more frequently in certain groups: people who drink too much alcohol are more likely to have dementia, caused either by the brain damage that results from the excess drinking or because of the associated vitamin deficiencies that many alcoholics suffer from. On the other hand, there is some evidence emerging that drinking alcohol, in moderation, especially red wine, may have a protective effect! However, as the commonest cause of dementia is Alzheimer's disease, which does not show a particular affinity for any specific group of people, dementia in general would appear to affect men and women in roughly equal measure and not to be associated with any other particular sub-group. The socio-economic group to which a person with dementia belongs does, however, have one important effect upon the progression of the illness, since those from lower socio-economic groups are more likely to be admitted to hospital or an alternative institution for prolonged periods of care and for the management of intercurrent illness.

Where do people with dementia live?

It is commonly assumed that most people with severe dementia live in institutions, especially hospitals. Nothing is further from the truth. Most studies that have looked at this have discovered that only 15–20 per cent or less of people with dementia are living permanently in an institution, and that a large proportion of those who are, are living in old people's homes rather than geriatric hospitals. In the UK there is very little NHS accommodation specifically set aside for the care, whether long-term or short-term, of people with dementia. In recent years there has been a considerable increase in the amount of private accommodation available in residential homes, and to a greater extent nursing homes, for those afflicted with an illness causing dementia. The standards vary and great care must be taken when chosing a home, as discussed later in this book. Even some of the residential accommodation for the elderly mentally infirm provided by local authorities is of an inadequate standard, in terms of architectural design, staffing ratios and inadequate training of the staff employed. This situation is, however, increasingly being addressed but, nevertheless, this is still an area of considerable concern to many of us.

There is little specialized accommodation and also a dearth of other facilities for younger sufferers with dementia; many of them are expected to be cared for alongside older patients with dementia and this of course causes many problems both for the sufferers and for the carers. In consequence, many relatives of younger sufferers soldier on at home despite the fact that it is made more difficult because of other commitments – to teenage children, for example. More interest by central government and the statutory services about the special needs of younger people with dementia, and their families, is long overdue but, like everything else, is mainly hampered by a lack of resources.

In general, elderly people with dementia are two and a half times more likely to be admitted to a hospital or other institution, and having got there to stay about six times as long, as other elderly people who do not have dementia. It is also more likely that an elderly man with dementia will be admitted to somewhere where he can be cared for, than a woman. It can be seen, however, that this is very similar to the general pattern among elderly people, in that there are far more elderly women living on their own than there are men.

Dementia is a common reason for people admitted to hospital as a result of some other disease, pneumonia or a heart attack say, to have their discharge delayed. Often this is because all concerned, both those outside in the community who are looking after them and those responsible for their care in the hospital, don't feel that they should go back to live alone; as a result they may spend a long time waiting for a place to become available in alternative accommodation – usually a social services welfare home (often specifically set aside for the elderly mentally infirm) or a private nursing home.

As already mentioned, the majority of people with dementia are living at home and it is the responsibility of the society in which we live to make it as easy as possible for those who wish to look after them to continue to do so. People with dementia have the same right as other people to live in their own home for as long as possible, even until they die. Often it is the anxieties and worries of those around them, rather than the financial implications, that lead to their admission to an institution.

As well as the community resources that are generally well known, it is also possible to make good use of hospital facilities to help support and maintain a person with dementia in the community. This will probably become the pattern more and more as time goes on. It is also heartening to note that despite beliefs to the contrary the younger generations today look after their elders as well as, if not better than, at any time in the past. The generalization that families do not care for their elders is untrue. There is little doubt that the quality, even if not the duration, of life is very likely to be better for old people, whether they have dementia or not, if they are allowed to live at home or in as normal a family environment as possible. The concept of community care, as long as it is supported by adequate hospital back-up, probably represents the best way forward as far as those with dementia are concerned, and may also be most cost-effective. In this context it is disturbing to see the move away from the provision of respite care by hard-pressed NHS Health Trusts. The excuse is often given that hospitals are there for the delivery of medical care rather than social care, but it is frequently impossible to separate the two, especially in relation to the needs of elderly people. A short-term respite admission that may provide much needed relief for a relative will often afford the opportunity for a demented patient's other medical problems to be assessed and treatment adjusted as necessary. This is more difficult to achieve in the context of a residential or nursing home. Thankfully, most Health Trusts accept the fact that there is the need for a small number of respite care beds and hopefully this will continue to be the case.

3

Diagnosis of the Conditions that Cause Dementia

Dementia provides two important diagnostic challenges. The first of these is the need to establish whether or not, in an elderly person, what appears to be an exaggeration of the normal mental changes of ageing is really dementia. The second involves determining the nature of the underlying illness if the presence of dementia is confirmed.

This chapter will provide an outline of the procedures involved and will also give some information about many of the more important conditions, both remediable and unremediable. As Alzheimer's disease, Lewy body dementia and vascular dementia are the three most common causes, and much is known about them that will be of interest to those caring for sufferers, each has a chapter of its own and is not discussed in detail here.

It is probably unnecessary for most readers to refer to the sections dealing with each of the different underlying illnesses – it may be less confusing to refer only to that condition which is affecting the person for whom they are caring. Professional carers – those working in old people's homes, nursing homes or with patients in their own homes – may find it helpful to read this section in its entirety, or to refer to it from time to time as necessary.

Confirming the presence of dementia

It has already been mentioned that dementia is separate from the acute confusional state caused by an intercurrent acute illness such as pneumonia, a urinary tract infection or the side-effects of drugs. These conditions are usually marked by a sudden onset rather than the more slow and gradual onset of dementia. Careful inquiry from a relative, friend or other person who knows the person under investigation well will help determine this and also whether there are any other current medical problems that make an acute confusional state more likely. An example of the latter is the repeated bouts of pneumonia to which people with chronic bronchitis, particularly heavy smokers, are prone. There are, however, many other medical conditions that can be responsible and unravelling these is best left to the general practitioner or, if necessary, a doctor in hospital.

Mrs Smith

A woman of seventy-three was admitted to the casualty department of a hospital at three in the morning one bitterly cold January night. She was brought in by the police, who had been alerted by her neighbours, in whose garden she had been found wandering in a confused and dishevelled state wearing nothing but a thin nightgown.

Mrs Smith, as we will call the patient, lived alone and was too confused and muddled to be able to answer any of the doctors' or the nurses' questions. She had no close relatives but appeared to be a respected and active member of the local community. Like many people of her age she had been noted to be becoming a little more forgetful on occasions, but nothing out of the ordinary.

The doctors examined her but were unable to find very much that was wrong. They therefore had to rely upon routine tests to try to discover the nature of her illness. An X-ray of her chest revealed that she had pneumonia even though there were no signs of this on stethoscope examination. In addition, testing her blood showed that the level of sugar was much higher than it should be. Mrs Smith was therefore considered to have diabetes and a chest infection.

The following morning the hospital managed to make contact with her next-door neighbours. They confirmed that they knew her quite well, and had noticed that for about a week she had been thirstier than usual. Otherwise, apart from seeming a little muddled the day before she was admitted to hospital, they had noticed nothing amiss.

This confirmed the impression of the hospital doctors that Mrs Smith had previously undiagnosed diabetes and that this was complicated by a chest infection. Both the diabetes and the pneumonia were sufficient cause for her to have become acutely confused and it didn't appear, from what her neighbours had said, that she had a progressive dementing illness.

Treatment for her diabetes and her pneumonia resulted in a dramatic improvement and after a fortnight she was back home just as well as she had been before her admission to hospital.

It is important to realize that even a person with a long history of dementia may also be the subject of an acute confusional state, as they may also develop an infection or other illness. This has to be considered when the person with dementia suddenly appears to get worse.

Mr Brown

Mrs Jones had been looking after her father, Mr Brown, who had been suffering with Alzheimer's disease for several years. He and her mother had lived in their own old people's bungalow until she had died. Mrs Jones was consulting her doctor to seek some treatment for her father because he had become more agitated and aggressive during the last week. Their general practitioner, however, declined to prescribe any form of treatment until he had had the opportunity of examining Mr Brown, and he arranged to call later that day. When he examined him, he discovered that her father's abdomen was much more swollen than it ought to have been and that it was tender and uncomfortable. It appeared that this was because the bladder was unable to drain its contents because of an obstruction caused by enlargement of the prostate gland, not uncommon in elderly men. The doctor therefore arranged for a catheter (a tube) to be inserted via the penis into the bladder, allowing it to drain. When he was relieved of the discomfort caused by his distended bladder, Mrs Jones' father became his normal self again and did not require any form of medication for his disturbed behaviour.

It can be very difficult to be certain whether the apparent early signs of dementia are really abnormal or whether the person concerned just has more marked age-related memory loss than most other people. There is no definite cut-off point between the effects of normal ageing and the onset of dementia and it is probable that, even if there were, it would differ in different individuals. The only way to be certain is to compare a person's intellectual ability with what he or she has been like in the past and unless there is a reliable estimate of this it can be very difficult. For this reason many doctors prefer to observe the person with a suspected, rather than a definite, dementia, over a period of time to see whether there is any further deterioration in intellectual ability of the sort that is typical of dementia. This will often mean that the person concerned will have to undergo careful memory testing and assessments of other aspects of mental function – often undertaken by a psychologist. A lot of the tests are administered nowadays with the help of a computer, which often makes them easier for the subject and more reliable for the psychologist. At the same time the doctor will need to have accurate information from a close relative or friend, if one exists, about any changes they have noticed in the person's ability to cope with day-to-day life over the same period.

As well as investigating different aspects of memory function, such as memory for recent events, events that have happened many years ago, and language memory, the tests may cover other areas including assessment of concentration, the ability to carry out simple calculations, the ability to draw or copy geometric shapes, and to identify simple objects, for example different types of coin held in the hand with the eyes closed. There are of course many other types of tests of intellectual function and in general they help to show whether a wide variety of different aspects of mental functioning are affected, even though this has not been suspected in the day-to-day life of the person suffering with possible early dementia. If there is indeed evidence to confirm suspicion of an early dementia, the pattern of the abnormal function may indicate which of the underlying causes is most likely, although it will rarely pinpoint a specific condition.

For a person in whom the abnormal mental functioning is more obvious and for whom the presence of dementia is unequivocal, the tests described above are often still necessary; they will help to determine the rate at which the disease is progressing if they are administered on more than one occasion over a period of time, and are also helpful in assessing the severity of the condition. Again, although some of the simple and short tests can be easily undertaken by a doctor or a nurse, if it is necessary to use the more complicated tests these are usually best administered by a psychologist, whose training allows him or her to assess and advise about such matters.

Diagnosing remediable conditions

The doctor's first and most important task is to make sure that there isn't a remediable cause for the dementia. This may be found in about one person in thirty who develops a dementing illness when he or she is over the age of seventy, and about one person in ten under this age. Discovering a treatable condition does not always cure the dementia; in some circumstances it merely stops it getting worse. For this reason it is important that the treatable causes are looked for as early in the course of the disease as possible. The types of illness that one finds vary from simple things like vitamin deficiencies, infections that have been quietly rumbling on for many years, malfunctioning of the thyroid gland, and abnormalities of the levels of different salts in the blood to more complicated things such as blood clots in the head that can be removed. It is often possible for the doctor to get some clue as to whether or not one of these conditions is present, but not infrequently there may be no outward sign that the person who is being investigated has anything abnormal wrong with him or her.

The most important vitamin deficiencies are probably those of the B group, including too little of vitamin B12 or B1. Folic acid is a related substance, a deficiency of which can also cause a reversible dementia, although this particular problem isn't encountered very often.

A very important condition not to miss is *normal pressure hydrocephalus*. This is in some ways similar to the problem that affects the brain in some children with spina bifida and results from an increased build-up of CSF in the hollow spaces (ventricles) within the brain. It may occur in people who have previously had a cerebral haemorrhage, a severe head injury sufficient to knock them out, or meningitis, but in many people there is no obvious predisposing cause. It can often be seen easily on a brain scan.

Normal pressure hydrocephalus has certain distinguishing features that will be apparent even to a lay person. Although many sufferers with dementia, whatever the underlying cause, become incontinent and have difficulty in walking, these usually feature later on towards the middle or later stages of their illness. In normal pressure hydrocephalus the incontinence and walking difficulties occur much earlier. To begin with the abnormal mental function often appears to be at least partly manifested by a slowness of thinking rather than an inability to think. The situation is not always clear-cut, however, and sometimes other causes of dementia can mimic normal pressure hydrocephalus; but if a person's symptoms are as described it is essential that the possibility of this diagnosis is investigated, and a brain scan is organized. The raised pressure can be treated by a small operation in which a fine tube has one of its ends placed within one of the hollow spaces, and the other into the chest or somewhere else into which the excess fluid can drain away, thus reducing the pressure within the brain.

In some people in whom dementia is suspected, the real cause of their illness is a different psychiatric condition, most commonly depression. It can often be very difficult to distinguish between depression and dementia, especially in older people. Sometimes the two conditions co-exist and then it can be very difficult to sort out the situation. For this reason many patients need to be seen by a psychiatrist. In some parts of the country psychiatrists are in any case responsible for assessing a person with dementia; in many places, however, this job is undertaken by other experts, either specialists in the care of the elderly or, especially for younger people, neurologists.

Another important condition that is to a certain extent treatable is the dementia associated with a high alcohol intake. This can occur for a number of reasons. On the one hand the alcohol itself can cause brain damage and on the other many people who are alcoholic have an inadequate diet and are therefore subject to vitamin and other dietary deficiencies. It has been shown that if a heavy drinker can change his or her habits, much of the damage that has occurred can be remedied.

It is fairly obvious from the range of treatable underlying conditions that may be present that a variety of tests will be needed. These are usually blood tests, which cause little if any upset to the person being investigated, collection of a sample of urine for investigation in some circumstances – and this can be a little more tricky – and sometimes a chest X-ray and an *electrocardiograph* (ECG), or heart tracing. In some cases it is necessary to arrange a lumbar puncture. This involves inserting a needle into the spinal canal through a gap between two of the bones that make up the spinal column. This procedure sometimes causes concern to a carer but with modern techniques a lumbar puncture is usually not traumatic, although it may be uncomfortable. The person suffering with dementia will usually not remember having undergone any of the tests, so if he or she has experienced some discomfort, it is soon forgotten. Testing can be important as sometimes it is the only way of being certain whether or not a treatable condition is present.

Lumbar punctures are not undertaken in very many cases; in situations where some years ago they would often have been necessary, a *brain scan*, often called a CT or CAT scan, will be arranged instead. Other types of scan that may be used include an MRI scan and a SPECT scan. An MRI scan is rather like a CT scan, i.e. it shows the structure of the brain. However, it can often show more detail than a CT scan. A SPECT scan is usually used to show the pattern of blood flow in the brain, which can help differentiate between some types of dementia. None of these scanning techniques is completely diagnostic. The scanners are only available in major centres and can only be used for a limited number of scans each day. It is not therefore possible for everybody with dementia to have a scan and the doctor has to use his common sense to decide which people most need one. Their application is discussed in a later chapter.

There are many treatable illnesses that can cause dementia although only a few people actually suffer with one or other of them. It is nevertheless extremely important to diagnose them when they are present and for this reason it is essential that anyone with dementia, or possible dementia, is investigated as early in the course of the disease as possible. Treatment may range from very simple measures such as replacing a vitamin deficiency, giving a tablet to replace a hormone that a failed thyroid gland can no longer produce, or treating a grumbling infection with appropriate antibiotics, to more complicated procedures that involve an operation, albeit a relatively minor one. Below are two case histories that are fairly typical.

Sister Mary

Dr Johnson was called to see a nun who lived in a convent. It was apparent that she had been becoming more and more confused over a considerable period of time and although her fellow nuns wanted to carry on looking after her as long as they could, they were beginning to find it very difficult. After carefully inquiring into the history of her illness and other relevant medical matters, Dr Johnson examined his new patient very carefully. He discovered some abnormalities when examining sensation in her legs and wondered whether she had a treatable cause for her dementia. He therefore arranged the appropriate tests and also those for the other conditions that might be present even though he could find no sign of them.

The results of the investigations showed that the dementia was probably the result of a deficiency of vitamin B12. Dr Johnson arranged for the district nurse to administer some B12 injections and a month later he returned to the convent to see whether this had resulted in any recovery. Although Sister Mary was still confused, her condition was much improved. He continued to see her regularly over a period of several months, during which she improved further, although to only a limited extent. Nevertheless there was now no question of her having to leave the convent as the other nuns found her once more a pleasant and easy person to manage.

Mr Allan

Mr Allan, though in his late fifties, was a well-built and muscular ex-professional wrestler. He lived with his wife, who for some time had been increasingly worried about his progressive forgetfulness and behaviour which was sometimes rather odd. For this reason he had been investigated by his general practitioner, who thought that he was suffering with Alzheimer's disease. All the usual treatable conditions that could be excluded by arranging blood tests had been proved to be absent; Mrs Allan was resigned to the future and had joined the support group of her local branch of the Alzheimer's Disease Society. About nine months after the diagnosis of Alzheimer's disease had been made she noticed that her husband was having episodes of incontinence, which she put down to the difficulty that he had begun to experience with walking, especially trying to get up and down the stairs.

Talking to her new friends in the support group she discovered that this wasn't similar to the experience of many of the others and so she went to her doctor to ask him why it was that her husband had developed difficulty with walking, and apparently also incontinence, at such an early stage in his condition. The general practitioner referred her husband for a second opinion and a brain scan was organized which showed that he had normal pressure hydrocephalus. A shunt (a fine tube) was inserted into the hollow space within his right hemisphere and the excess fluid allowed to drain off into his chest. Six weeks later he was considerably improved, no longer incontinent, able to walk normally, and with a considerable degree of improvement in his mental function. The latter continued to progress, but he never quite regained the intellectual ability that he had enjoyed before his illness began.

Unremediable causes of dementia

Some of the conditions that cause dementia, which at the moment are untreatable in the sense of being incurable, are described briefly in the pages that follow for the benefit of people who have a relative suffering with one of these illnesses. The following pages should also enable those who work with many dementia sufferers, and who therefore may come across a variety of different underlying conditions, to obtain a general overview of some of the less common disorders that are responsible for this type of intellectual breakdown.

Pick's disease and similar conditions, e.g. fronto-temporal dementia

Pick's disease was described in 1892, before Alzheimer's disease, but appears to occur much less frequently. Like Alzheimer's disease it is a chronic degenerative condition of the brain. In the majority of cases it appears as if there is an inherited tendency and it strikes particularly in late middle age, i.e. in general at a younger age than Alzheimer's disease. It is said to affect women a little more frequently than men.

The most striking feature of this condition is the way in which the degeneration and wasting of the brain tissue appear to be confined to two lobes in particular, the frontal and temporal lobes. Sometimes the left hemisphere appears to be more affected than the right and the disease also seems to start at the front end of these lobes. When one examines the brain under the microscope there is a considerable degree of nerve cell loss and also an increase in the numbers of the non-nerve cell population, the *glia*, in the outer layers of the brain – the cortex. Some of the neurones are distorted in a particular fashion; the nerve cell bodies appear to be distended by some abnormal material that has collected within the cell.

The symptoms that a patient shows reflect the site at which the damage occurs. Abnormalities of the frontal lobe often result in deterioration in personality and disorders of mood. These changes make it quite clear that something is amiss, especially as they usually occur in a younger person. Unlike some of the other illnesses that cause dementia, in the early stages of the disease memory function and the ability to use language are less affected in proportion to the personality and mood changes. In many instances therefore it is possible to suspect the diagnosis after questioning a relative or close friend and examining the person concerned. A brain scan may then show that the atrophy has particularly affected the frontal and temporal lobes and this makes the diagnosis almost certain. In most of the other dementias memory function is affected first and is usually one of the aspects of mental function that is affected most.

The condition is not always easy to spot, however, and can sometimes mimic the commoner illnesses such as Alzheimer's disease. Alzheimer's sufferers may be caught shoplifting because they have absent-mindedly put an article in their bag, forgetting that they ought to pay for it. Rather than having forgotten, Pick's sufferers may well have felt that they should not be expected to pay or perhaps just wanted to see if they could get away with not doing so.

As the disease progresses it becomes more and more difficult to distinguish from other conditions like Alzheimer's. Often the diagnosis is only made when the brain is examined after the person has died. Most people with Pick's disease live for five to ten years after the diagnosis has been made, sometimes a little longer.

We now know that there are a number of different conditions that specifically affect the frontal and temporal lobes, and that Pick's disease is just one of these. For this reason people with dementia affecting these lobes of the brain are sometimes referred to as having a 'fronto-temporal dementia'. This is because it is often difficult, while the sufferer is alive, to be sure which of the conditions is damaging the brain in any particular individual unless there are some very definite clues, for example if another member of the family has had a similar illness and Pick's disease has been diagnosed at autopsy.

Huntington's chorea

Huntington's chorea is a very complicated disorder of the brain. In most families it is inherited in what is known as a *dominant autosomal pattern*. This means that approximately half the children of an affected parent will suffer with the condition, which usually strikes in middle age or early old age. It therefore poses quite an ethical problem, as a potential sufferer cannot know that he or she will definitely develop the condition until the time for having children is past. Genetic testing often means we are able to determine accurately whether or not a person from an affected family is going to develop the disease, and anyone who is so diagnosed will immediately know what the future holds for them and can plan accordingly. As the reader will be able to imagine, genetic testing is fraught with emotional complications and it is essential that genetic counselling is available before a person agrees to have the test. Some people would prefer not to know, rather than live with the certain knowledge that they are going to die from an unpleasant and progressive disease later in life. On the other hand, some potential sufferers feel a need to be informed of their own risk, so that they can plan their lives accordingly. This is a very individual decision and skilled counselling is essential to help each person make the right decision for him or her. Once the decision has been made, further counselling is often necessary to help the person come to terms with the consequences of their new knowledge, or lack of it.

The disease tends to start in middle age with abnormal movements of the limbs, which usually worsen over the years; at the same time dementia sets in. People suffering with Huntington's chorea may also be afflicted by other psychiatric conditions, the most common of which is probably depression.

Most of the damage from Huntington's chorea falls on some of the deep-lying areas of grey matter, especially a structure called the *caudate nucleus* which lies in the outside wall of the main ventricle. Cells are also lost from the cerebral cortex and there are changes in the brain's biochemistry.

A brain scan will show that the ventricles have increased in size, especially that part that lies adjacent to the caudate nucleus. It is the shrinkage of the caudate nucleus that is partly responsible for the increase in the ventricular size.

Some of the abnormal movements, technically described as

chorea, hence the name, can be reduced with special drugs, but none of these are of any help in treating the dementia itself.

Creutzfeldt-Jakob disease

Creutzfeldt-Jakob disease (CJD) is probably a collection of different clinical syndromes, or patterns of disease presentation, which have in common the same transmissible causal agent. That is, they may be caused by infection from one individual to another. The infection can even be transmitted by using on one patient neurosurgical instruments that have been earlier used in an operation on another patient suffering with this condition, despite the instruments having been sterilized in the normal manner between operations. For this reason great care is now taken of the instruments when a person who may have CJD is being operated on.

It should be stressed, however, that this condition is very rare, which means that it must be a very difficult disease to transmit from one person to another; there is no evidence of anyone developing CJD as a result of caring for someone with the disease. Nevertheless, those who are working with or looking after a sufferer from CJD should take seriously the precautions advised by the doctors in charge.

The disease is accompanied by a pathological process that causes lots of what appear to be microscopic 'holes' within the substance of the brain. It is marked in most cases by a particularly rapid progression of dementia associated with abnormalities of movement. Unlike Huntington's chorea, the movement problem is more a case of difficulty in maintaining balance and co-ordination than the development of extra abnormal movements, with the exception of 'twitches', which occur in most sufferers from both diseases. These are called *myoclonic jerks*. The physical manifestations of the disease are very variable, depending upon which structures in the brain are particularly affected.

CJD usually runs its course in three to twelve months, but in some cases it is much more prolonged. As with the other chronic conditions that cause dementia there is no diagnostic test although often one is helped, albeit late in the disease, by an *electro-encephalograph* (EEG) picture, showing up an abnormality.

'Mad Cow Disease'

All readers will be aware of the new form of CJD that appears to be linked to 'Mad Cow Disease', more correctly known as Bovine Spongiform Encephalopathy. This is the disease of cows, thought to be contracted by their having been fed with contaminated foodstuffs, possibly food containing material from sheep affected by a condition known as Scrapie. The new form of CJD, which particularly affects younger people, appears to be linked to BSE and may be contracted by having eaten meat from affected animals. The number of cases identified so far is very small, and although some experts have prophesied that there will be a gradual increase in the numbers of people affected by this disorder, at the time of writing there is no convincing evidence that an epidemic is beginning. Nevertheless, only time will tell. The risk of further infection in humans is becoming increasingly smaller as precautions to remove affected animals from the food chain have been enforced now for a considerable period of time.

Parkinson's disease

It used to be said that about a third of people with Parkinson's disease would eventually develop dementia. This view would nowadays be considered controversial. Parkinson's disease can affect the intellect, but in many instances this is insufficient to cause what we would consider to be dementia. It is particularly associated with a slowness of thinking and reacting, but often memory is relatively intact until the later stages in those whose intellect ultimately fails.

It is important not to forget that most people who develop Parkinson's disease are relatively elderly and are therefore also likely to develop other conditions that occur more frequently in older people, illnesses that cause dementia among them. This has muddied the waters, and it is probable that some people whose dementia has been ascribed to their Parkinson's disease were all the time suffering from some other unrelated condition, also causing dementia. Taking account of this possibility, a more accurate representation of the truth would probably be that only about one person in ten who has Parkinson's disease is likely to develop dementia because of the Parkinson's disease itself. The total number of people with Parkinson's disease and dementia will be more than one in ten, as some of them may also have Alzheimer's disease, vascular dementia or some other cause. It is probable that some people who were previously diagnosed as suffering from Parkinson's disease and dementia, or Alzheimer's disease with some of the signs of Parkinsonism, may really have been suffering with a Lewy body dementia (see chapter 6).

It should also be understood that some of the medicines that are given to people with Parkinson's disease to treat their movement disorders may themselves cause confusion. If a person with Parkinson's is found to be confused, rather than immediately attributing this to dementia caused by the disease it is important first to make sure that it isn't a side-effect of the sufferer's drugs.

Cerebral tumours

A cerebral tumour can cause dementia. Such tumours can be divided into two types – primary and secondary. Primary cerebral tumours are those that arise within the brain whereas secondary tumours spread there from a site somewhere else in the body, usually arriving via the bloodstream. Secondary tumours arise when a few cells from a tumour, say a cancer of the breast, are taken by the bloodstream and planted as seeds in the brain, where they grow and destroy brain tissue. Sometimes there are many small secondary deposits. They may cause all sorts of other symptoms and side-effects and don't always cause dementia. Since most brain tumours are unsuitable for X-ray therapy or surgical removal, it is usually only possible to treat the symptoms, such as headache. However, some primary tumours, especially one called a *meningioma*, can often be completely and safely removed. A meningioma can grow to a very large size and still be removed. It is therefore another of the treatable conditions that can be diagnosed from a brain scan. In most tumours, unfortunately, although treatment can be given to improve the quality of life of the person concerned, the tumour will eventually be responsible for the patient's death.

AIDS and dementia

The majority of people with HIV, the virus infection that causes AIDS, do not develop a dementia, although some of them do develop more minor intellectual problems, for example difficulty with memory. Some AIDS sufferers, however, do develop a dementing illness which may have two different causes, either acting alone or sometimes in conjunction with each other. It is possible that the HIV virus itself may damage some parts of the brain, but in many other cases the dementia is caused by opportunistic infections which gain a foothold because of the body's lowered immunity. Sometimes tumours can also contribute to this process.

Dementia associated with AIDS is usually, as one would expect, a condition that affects younger people, but just occasionally this diagnosis is raised as a possibility in an older person, albeit very rarely.

Who is responsible for making the diagnosis?

Well, who is responsible for making the diagnosis? The answer is that we all have an important part to play: relatives, friends and sometimes people with dementia themselves. We all need to face up squarely to the possibility that someone we love or care for may be developing dementia. Unless we do so and arrange for them to see a doctor as early as possible, the illness causing the dementia, if it does indeed exist, may progress further during the period of inaction. This would be particularly important if the person who was the object of the concern were to have one of the treatable underlying causes.

The doctor that most people will see first is the general practitioner. He or she should be willing to listen carefully to the history of the apparent intellectual decline, should undertake a careful and complete examination, and arrange appropriate tests. In the first instance these will probably be the simple blood tests described earlier, undertaken in the hope that a treatable cause will be discovered. When a more complicated assessment is required, the general practitioner will usually refer the patient to a specialist, who may be a geriatrician, a psychiatrist specializing in diseases of the elderly, or a neurologist, depending upon the patient's age and other factors. These hospital specialists may extend the examination and arrange additional tests. They will often ask the psychologist, trained to assess intellectual function and behaviour, to help with the assessment. Often it will be necessary to repeat this after a period of time.

In some parts of the country there are special memory disorder clinics. They are staffed by doctors and psychologists, and others who are specially trained to detect dementia, even in its early stages, to try to diagnose the underlying cause, and to help plan ahead with the family if the condition is untreatable. Many patients attending a memory disorders clinic will have a physical, psychiatric, and psychological assessment – a very intensive programme.

Others who may be involved in helping to make the diagnosis include occupational therapists and specially trained psychiatric nurses who work in the community.

4

Alzheimer's Disease

Alois Alzheimer was a pathologist with a particular interest in the changes caused by diseases of the nervous system. Born in Bavaria in 1864, he studied medicine in three German universities – Würzburg, Tübingen, and Berlin – receiving his MD in 1887. At this stage he was working on the glands in the ear that produce ear-wax; it was later that he specialized in the pathology of brain diseases, eventually becoming professor and director of a large anatomical laboratory in Munich's highly regarded Neuro-Pathology Centre. In 1912 he moved to Breslau to become professor and also director of the Psychiatric and Neurological Institute there, where he was able to combine both clinical practice and research. He died in 1915 from heart and kidney failure.

Alzheimer published the first report of the disease that now bears his name in 1907. He examined the brain of a woman in her fifties who had been noted as having rapidly increasing difficulties with memory such that she became lost in her own home, carried objects about with her for no apparent purpose, and sometimes hid them. At times she screamed for no obvious reason and at others appeared to think that she was going to be murdered. Eventually she became totally helpless and had to be admitted to an institution. Whilst there she often wandered about aimlessly, complaining that she didn't understand why she was there or didn't know where she was. She called repeatedly

for her husband and daughter. Her mental deterioration progressed relentlessly and she died about five years after the disease
first started. At this stage she was totally helpless, practically
bed-bound, and mentally inaccessible to those around her.

When Alzheimer examined her brain he discovered strange
fibrillary material within some of the nerve cells, and collections
of abnormal material deposited in the form of disc-like plaques,
especially in the cortex.

Towards a better understanding

Traditionally the pre-senile dementias – those occurring before
the age of sixty-five – were considered to be caused by diseases
like Alzheimer's disease, Pick's disease, Huntington's chorea,
and so on, whereas those in older people were thought to be a
consequence of ageing of the brain or possibly arteriosclerosis.
This rather confused picture began to be corrected only in the
late 1960s and early 1970s when Professor, now Sir Martin,
Roth and his colleagues, including Professor Tomlinson and Dr
Blessed, examined the brains of a large series of normal old
people and also subjects with dementia. They showed quite
conclusively that Alzheimer's disease was the most common
cause of dementia in people of all ages, that the next most
common cause was dementia resulting from vascular disease,
and that in a small proportion of people these two conditions
occurred together. Interestingly, at that time they did not have
the technology to recognize the third common cause of dementia,
that is Lewy body dementia. Had they been able to recognize
this disorder, we would have known about its existence and
importance for much longer than has been the case.

Despite this knowledge about Alzheimer's disease, for many
years dementia in the elderly was still considered by many doctors
to be caused by hardening of the arteries and it wasn't until the
beginning of the 1980s that research into Alzheimer's disease
really began to gain momentum. A modicum of research was,

however, underway in the intervening years and important discoveries were made, including a description of some of the biochemical abnormalities that will be described later. Research into Alzheimer's really took off, however, in the mid-eighties and throughout the world all the latest techniques that are employed in medical research are now being focussed on this condition.

Symptoms

Most doctors think of Alzheimer's disease as being characterized by abnormalities of cortical function which they call *amnesia*, *aphasia* and *agnosia*. This is not as complicated as it sounds. The cortex is of course the outer layer of grey cells which lie on the surface of the brain and the three terms refer, respectively, to general memory failure, difficulty in remembering or understanding the names of objects, and failure to recognize people or objects. The overall symptoms are, however, very much more complicated than this and the disease often progresses along a different path in different individuals, although the later stages of the different courses of the disease tend to resemble each other. For this reason I am going to describe the symptoms caused by the malfunction of the three major lobes of the brain – the temporal lobe, the frontal lobe and the parietal lobe – although there is some overlap in the relationship between structure and function.

Temporal lobe changes

This is the part of the brain that appears to bear the brunt of the disease process and in many ways it often seems as if it is the seat of the abnormal changes which eventually spread out from here to involve the other structures. The earliest symptom of Alzheimer's disease is usually memory loss and it is the temporal lobe and in particular a special structure within it called the *hippocampus* that are particularly associated with memory. Memory is often divided into two types – classified as short-term and long-term memory by most people working in this field. It may be more accurate to use a slightly different concept, that of recent and remote memory. In this discussion recent or short-term memory will be used to refer to memory processes relating to the preceding hours or days, occasionally a little longer, while long-term or remote memory can go back as far as childhood.

The way in which memory is affected in Alzheimer's disease is, in the old trade-union manner, 'last in, first out'. A quite severely demented person, particularly with Alzheimer's disease, can often remember in detail activities that happened in childhood while having forgotten what he or she had for lunch, even though that may have been only half an hour earlier. Some people use short-term memory to refer to the type of memory that only lasts a few seconds and this also is severely affected.

It would seem as if memory normally works by transferring information from very short-term memory processes to longer-term memory processes and the major defect of Alzheimer's disease may be an inability to store any new information. Not only is it more difficult to put it into the long-term memory store, but once there it doesn't seem to last as long as information that was put there years before.

The consequence of this memory problem is the familiar picture of a sufferer from Alzheimer's disease being unable to grasp what is said to him or her, needing to have items repeated, needing to write lists, forgetting to keep appointments, and so on. This can often lead to hazards in the home and as the dementing process advances it is not unknown for relatives to discover that saucepans are put on the stove and allowed to boil dry, or gas taps turned on but not lit.

An example of this kind of behaviour is the person suffering with Alzheimer's disease who went shopping in a nearby town, having driven ten miles from the village in which he lived. After completing as many of the purchases as he could remember and having got into difficulty in working out the change, he then set out to find his car to make the return journey home. Unfortunately, he could not find his car anywhere, decided it had been stolen, and managed to walk all the way home, turning up several hours late, having caused much distress to his wife. This example illustrates two aspects of memory. On the one hand he was unable to remember where he had parked his car, which was in fact only about thirty seconds' walk from the store in which he had done most of his shopping; on the other hand the long journey home was sufficiently familiar to enable him to arrive safely back, although rather late. When questioned he said that he hadn't been able to telephone his wife as he couldn't remember their telephone number and he hadn't been able to take a bus because he couldn't remember the name of the village in which he lived; being unfamiliar with the bus service, he was unable to ask someone which bus he should take.

The pattern of memory loss, particularly the differentiation between very short-term (lasting only a few seconds) and longer but still relatively recent memory function, changes as the disease progresses, with the very short-term memory traces becoming more disturbed as the disease advances, whereas early on in the condition it is memory loss over a period of a few minutes or so that is most marked.

Doctors often try to test memory by asking questions that test the subjects' ability to place themselves in the correct environment – space or time. The former is particularly affected by the context in which the question is asked. For instance questioning an Alzheimer's disease sufferer after he or she has been moved to a hospital, clinic, or ward will frequently reveal disorientation in space, while the same question asked of him or her at home may elicit the correct answer.

Frontal lobe changes

The frontal lobe is the part of the brain that controls certain aspects of our personality, particularly keeping our behaviour in check. Some forms of frontal lobe damage will lead to uninhibited behaviour, for example when a person has drunk too much alcohol. It seems as if alcohol is a stimulant, but in fact it depresses those parts of the frontal lobe that control behaviour, releasing inhibitions.

One of the features of Alzheimer's disease that is said to differentiate it from the dementia that is characteristic of vascular dementia is the change in personality often noticed in the Alzheimer's sufferer. This can take the form of being unusually irritable or apathetic, or showing a lack of concern about matters that would formerly have been of importance to them, such as the management of the family finances. In the early stages the subject may realize that forgetfulness is a problem, but it may cause no undue anxiety; in some cases, however, the realization may be accompanied by considerable anxiety. It is usually relatives or friends who are responsible for alerting the doctor to the fact that something is wrong. Sometimes mood is very unstable, with anger or tears suddenly appearing for no obvious reason. This, however, is also a feature of the dementia that is caused by vascular dementia. As the disease progresses, restless wandering may occur and later becomes particularly troublesome at night. Eventually there is an almost complete disintegration of personality, with a lack of interest in personal hygiene and standards of dress, and occasionally the development of unpleasant behavioural habits – including going to the toilet in inappropriate and embarrassing places.

Many sufferers with Alzheimer's disease lose things and accuse others of having stolen them. This paranoid behaviour sometimes progresses to the stage where it is imagined that others are plotting or planning against them, especially if there has been any talk of alternative accommodation. Hallucinations may also occur and these may take the form of the sufferer seeing people or objects that are not really there or, less occasionally, being told to do things by voices from uncertain sources.

As mentioned earlier, another feature of Alzheimer's disease is the development of difficulty with speech. Speech and language functions are controlled by special centres in different parts of the brain, not just the frontal lobe, but will be considered here for convenience.

The most important language disorder is difficulty with names. This can take two forms. The names of common objects may be forgotten so that when a pen is required, it will be referred to as 'that thing that you write with', and as the disease progresses even this way round the problem may not be possible, with the sufferer just pointing at an object and demanding that he or she be given it. Sometimes, however, a second type of difficulty with language occurs and this is not so much the naming of an object, but difficulty recognizing the name if used by somebody else.

There is a particular area of the left frontal lobe in most people that is responsible for the control of this aspect of language and this is affected early on in the course of Alzheimer's disease. Sometimes it isn't noticed in the very early stages unless careful tests are undertaken. However, once the language disorder has become marked, it usually indicates that the disease is going to progress more rapidly than hitherto. Generally, difficulty in using the name of an object occurs earlier in the disease whereas difficulty in understanding the name of an object when somebody else uses the word occurs later.

One further aspect of frontal lobe function that is often abnormal in the later stages of Alzheimer's disease is the reappearance of reflexes that are more typically found in young babies. If the palm of an infant is stroked with a finger, the finger will be seized. Because these reflexes occur early in life and disappear as the nervous system matures, they are referred to as *primitive reflexes*. When there is significant degeneration in the frontal lobes, the grasp reflexes and others reappear. Although they are occasionally present in apparently normal people throughout life, their presence in an Alzheimer's sufferer usually indicates quite an advanced stage in the disease.

Parietal lobe changes

The parietal lobe puts together all the information that our brains obtain in order to allow us to undertake quite complicated activities. For instance, one of the characteristic problems experienced relatively early in the course of Alzheimer's is difficulty with operating machinery or equipment such as a washing machine or television, and later with dressing. Difficulties like this, which are not caused by a specific abnormality in one of the nervous pathways outside the brain, are called *apraxias*. The presence of apraxias for a variety of activities may indicate that the disease is going to progress fairly rapidly.

The parietal lobe also integrates the information that is obtained from the senses. Most people will be able to distinguish between a ten pence piece and a fifty pence piece when put in their hand, even if their eyes are closed so that they can't see what the coin looks like. A person with parietal lobe damage won't be able to do this, and is said to be suffering from an *agnosia*.

A frequently employed test of parietal lobe function, which is really trying to elicit evidence of the presence of apraxia, is to ask the subject to draw or copy a diagram. This may be a simple clock-face or a more complicated structure such as intersecting geometric shapes.

Depression

The manner in which the symptoms of Alzheimer's disease occur in many people is complicated by the coexistence of depression. This is usually assumed to be a reaction to the disease – the result of patients realizing that something has gone seriously wrong with the way in which their mind works. This may well be an over-simplification because we know that some of the biochemical changes in the brain that are found in Alzheimer's disease are similar to those that are found in the brain of people with depression. These biochemical changes may occur in the Alzheimer brain when the person concerned did not appear to be depressed while alive. It may also be that in some people these depression-like biochemical changes are sufficiently severe to result in depression. As the disease progresses, the depression will often lift. Doctors have to be very careful if they try to treat an Alzheimer's disease sufferer for depression since many of the older drugs that are used can actually make memory function worse.

Depression may also mimic a dementia, including Alzheimer's disease. If there is any doubt about the nature of the depressive symptoms, careful assessment by a psychiatrist is essential and sometimes a trial of treatment is also needed.

Tests of intellectual function

Alzheimer's disease is probably the most difficult of the dementing illnesses to distinguish from the changes of normal ageing. As mentioned before, there is indeed some degree of memory impairment in many people as they grow older although this may not be as great as was once imagined. As the earliest sign of Alzheimer's disease is often exaggerated memory loss, there is often a grey area in the interpretation of tests of memory function. It is therefore often necessary to test memory function on successive occasions over several months before one can be certain whether or not Alzheimer's disease is present.

There are many tests of intellectual function; some are very long and complicated and others are simple and quick. As one might expect, the shorter and simpler the test, the more likely it is that the information will be unhelpful or inaccurate. Nevertheless, because of the time involved, the initial tests often have to be the short and simple ones. Many of these are employed by district nurses, health visitors and doctors when they first meet a person with suspected dementia. The tests usually involve a few questions that are designed to test different types of memory function – the ability to use language correctly and parietal lobe function. The performance of more complicated tasks such as the ability to carry out simple calculations may also be examined. In many ways these are most useful if the results are normal. An abnormal result will not diagnose dementia; on the contrary, it will indicate that something is wrong and that further assessment is required. In difficult cases the patient will need to be referred to a qualified psychologist who will perform the more extensive and sensitive tests. These will usually go a long way towards determining whether or not dementia is present, and may also provide information that will help in deciding which condition may be causing the dementia.

Nowadays many of these tests have been put on to computer; colourful images on a television screen help to keep the attention of the person being tested and reduce the opportunity for inaccurate responses to creep in because of adverse interactions between the patient and the person doing the testing.

The structural changes in the brain

Loss of brain tissue – atrophy of the brain substance – leads to a progressive shrinkage of the brain as the disease advances. Viewed externally, the brain therefore looks smaller and the spaces or *sulci* between the ridges, *gyri*, become bigger. Internally, the hollow spaces within the brain enlarge; the brain from a person with Alzheimer's disease weighs less than normal. The degree of wasting is most marked in younger patients; in many older people with this disease the brain can appear very similar to that of a non-demented elderly person. The shape and degree of wasting of the brain can be seen on modern brain scans.

Although there is no particular diagnostic feature of Alzheimer's disease when the brain changes are observed in this way, the absence of any other abnormality, a cerebral tumour or stroke-damage for example, makes the diagnosis of Alzheimer's disease more likely. The similarity, however, between the degree of brain wasting in normal old people and elderly subjects with Alzheimer's makes this observation of less value than in younger people, for whom any significant degree of atrophy is quite clearly abnormal. The most marked loss of brain substance usually occurs in the temporal lobes, including the structure known as the hippocampus. As this part of the brain is particularly important for memory function, this fits in well with our knowledge that memory loss is one of the major symptoms of the disease. Considerable research effort is presently being employed to try and improve our understanding of the structural changes in the brain that occur in Alzheimer's disease, in the hope that this will enable brain scans to assist with earlier diagnosis, and some progress is indeed being made in this field.

At a microscopic level there are two main changes, both of which have already been briefly mentioned. One of these is the formation of disc-like plaques of abnormal tissue, found especially in the grey matter of the cortex; the other is the collection inside nerve cells of bundles of an abnormal fibril-like substance, *neurofibrillary tangles*. Both of these occur to a lesser extent in the normal ageing brain. In Alzheimer's disease the changes are more widespread and greater in number.

Further changes that are found in the brain of a person suffering from Alzheimer's disease include abnormalities within the cells and the formation, within the walls of some of the small blood vessels, of an abnormal substance called *amyloid*. This amyloid is very similar to the material that is found in the centre of the plaques. It is found in significant amounts in many cases of Alzheimer's disease and is also sometimes discovered in apparently normal older people.

Amyloid is found in other parts of the body in other medical conditions. Some researchers have looked for a connection between the amyloid of other conditions and that of Alzheimer's disease. The amyloid of Alzheimer's is very different to that found in, say, the liver or the heart in other unrelated illnesses. At the moment it seems unlikely that there is any specific link.

The abnormalities that affect the brain cells would seem to lead to the death of many of them. Therefore when the cerebral cortex is examined under the microscope it becomes apparent that there are, in many areas, fewer cells than there should be and that a significant proportion of those that remain are affected by abnormal changes such as neurofibrillary tangle formation. In addition, some of the supporting or glial cells increase in number. The general pattern of these changes, however, varies considerably from case to case and the largest number of nerve cells appears to be lost from the temporal lobe and the hippocampus. The actual degree of cell loss is still a matter of dispute because measurement of cell numbers in the brain is technically very difficult. It is, however, generally agreed that greatest cell loss occurs in younger subjects.

There are also changes in the pattern and extent of branching of the nerve fibres in the brain. Although these are difficult to understand, they are probably one of the more important changes as nerve cells interact with each other via the connections, or synapses, made between their nerve fibres and the nerve fibres of other cells. The disruption of this system of communication leads to neurological disorders.

The plaques, commonly called *senile plaques*, and neurofibrillary tangles are the best-researched of the abnormalities and probably the most important.

Senile plaques

Senile plaques can be shown to consist of granular material in the centre of which is a substance loosely referred to as the *core*. The granular material on the rim of the plaque consists largely of nerve cell fibres, their contents, and a collection of glial cells.

In other words, this rim consists largely of components that are normally part of brain cells. The centre of the plaque is made out of amyloid, now known to be similar to the amyloid protein found in some of the blood vessels.

These plaques multiply in the cerebral cortex in normal people as they age and are occasionally discerned in the brains of intellectually normal people in their thirties and forties. More usually, however, they begin to build up after the age of fifty. In a person with Alzheimer's disease they are present in considerably increased numbers and in some cases it is difficult to find an area where you can see the normal structure of the cortex because there are so many plaques crowded into the grey matter. Although they look like flat structures, this is because they are normally observed in cross-section. In fact, they are spherical or oval and seeing them on a microscope slide is rather like taking a hard-boiled egg, cutting a thin slice out of it, laying it down, and looking at it. The yolk would be the equivalent of the amyloid core and the white around it the equivalent of the rim of granular material.

In Alzheimer's disease these plaques particularly affect those parts of the brain that are associated with memory function. They spread to involve heavily all the grey matter, but not the white matter – that part of the brain that is predominantly made up of nerve fibres.

It seems very much as if the plaques are composed of nerve cells that have begun to degenerate, glial cells that may have been attracted towards the degenerating nerve cell structures, and the amyloid substance in the centre. How they are formed is a matter of conjecture. One theory is that the protein that makes up the amyloid core leaks out of damaged blood vessels, although this theory is beginning to seem less likely; another is that abnormal processes within nerve cells lead to the death of some of their branches and that this somehow leads to the formation of plaques.

Amyloid is also deposited in more diffuse plaques in between the nerve cells and fibres, as well as in the more typical senile plaque described above. In experimental conditions we know that amyloid can damage brain cells, and one theory is that the amyloid that is deposited in this more diffuse fashion damages the surrounding structures, eventually leading to the formation of the more typical Alzheimer's disease plaque described above.

Neurofibrillary tangles

Neurofibrillary tangles occur inside brain cells, particularly the larger neurones. Again, they are especially seen in those parts of the brain that are involved in memory function and like plaques are present in small numbers, in circumscribed areas of the brain, in people who are old but intellectually normal. Eventually the cells containing them die and all one can see is the neurofibrillary tangle material lying free in the brain substance – usually cortical grey matter. Each of these tangles is made up of lots of smaller filaments arranged in a helix or spiral. They are mainly situated in the cell body, but may extend into some of the nerve cell processes. Many people feel that neurofibrillary tangles are a better indicator of the presence of Alzheimer's disease than is the presence of plaques. The numbers of tangles, rather like the number of plaques, relates well to the severity of the dementia, people with more severe Alzheimer's disease usually having greater numbers of both.

The cause of neurofibrillary tangle formation is, like so many aspects of Alzheimer's disease, still a matter of speculation. It has been thought that aluminium may be responsible, but, for reasons discussed in a later chapter, this seems unlikely. It may be that there is a genetic cause or that some infectious agent is responsible. At the moment we really don't know, but a better understanding of the processes that lead to the formation of tangles may well help us in the fight against the disease.

The biochemical changes in the brain

Knowledge of the biochemical abnormalities in the brain in other neurological conditions, especially Parkinson's disease, has led to attempts at treatment that have been at least partially successful. Abnormalities in the biochemistry of the Alzheimer brain have therefore been studied in some detail, with the first important finding being reported in the mid-1970s. This was an abnormality in the chemical messenger or neurotransmitter system that uses a substance called *acetylcholine* to switch on different nerve cells in the message chain. Acetylcholine itself is difficult to measure and so other chemicals intimately related to its biochemistry have been studied instead, giving an indirect indication of the changes in the acetylcholine neurotransmitter system. It has been known for some time now that there is a deficiency of acetylcholine in cases of Alzheimer's. The acetylcholine system is particularly important for memory function so again the changes found in the brain relate very closely to the symptoms that patients with Alzheimer's disease suffer.

During the last ten years, abnormalities have also been found in many other neurotransmitter systems and this probably explains the multiplicity of symptoms and signs that people who develop Alzheimer's disease display. These biochemical abnormalities, usually in the form of a lack of the neurotransmitter chemicals, are more marked in younger patients; in some older people with Alzheimer's disease the only significant abnormality may well be the lack of acetylcholine.

These neurotransmitter substances are broadly classified into two groups, depending upon whether they are made within the cortex – the outer rim of grey matter in the brain – or in other areas of grey matter buried more deeply within the brain, from where they are transported along nerve fibres into the cortex. Those that are formed within the cortex itself are known as the *intrinsic neurotransmitters* and the others are called the *extrinsic neurotransmitters*. We now know that the intrinsic neurotransmitters are largely unaffected, and that the major abnormalities lie within the brain cell systems that use the extrinsic neurotransmitters. Acetylcholine is an extrinsic neuro-transmitter as are two others, *noradrenaline* and *serotonin* (5.HT). Acetylcholine is the most severely affected.

The most important site in which acetylcholine is made lies in the base of the brain in a very small ribbon of cells called the *basal nucleus*. Noradrenaline and serotonin are made in collections of grey matter within the brain-stem. When these areas are examined carefully through the microscope it can be seen that they, like the cerebral cortex, are also abnormal. There appears to be a loss of cells and many of the cells that remain contain neurofibrillary tangles. Plaques may also be present. When this was discovered, some researchers thought that perhaps the major abnormality in Alzheimer's disease lay in these deeper-lying structures (the base of the brain and the brain-stem), and that the changes elsewhere were secondary. This is still a matter for speculation, but most researchers now believe that the primary change is probably in the cortex, and that the changes in the other structures are secondary to cortical damage.

Genes and Alzheimer's disease

It has been known for some time that Alzheimer's disease is inherited in some families. By and large this is mainly restricted to some of those people who develop Alzheimer's disease at an early age, for example in their fifties and early sixties. The family history is easy to recognize as the disease usually presents itself in a similar way in a particular family. The pattern varies in different families. However, it has to be said that there are some families where individuals do develop the disease in surprisingly different ways.

This inheritance is caused by abnormalities in genes. The genes are chemical structures that are contained within larger structures known as the *chromosomes*. Chromosomes are themselves concentrated in a special structure called the *nucleus* which lies in the centre of the cell. The genes act as a blue-print and control the way in which all the cells in our body work, and also all our characteristics. They are rather like an architect's plan and in the body will determine some quite obvious features of our make-up, for example the colour of our eyes, the colour of our hair, whether we have difficulty with putting on weight, and many other features, many of which are hidden within the biochemical processes that take place within our cells and organs.

Genes often work in conjunction with environmental factors and the way in which a person develops may result from an interplay between the genetic blue-print and external influences that may modify genetically controlled processes. Most of the cells in our body contain forty-six chromosomes, that is twenty-three pairs, and each pair is numbered such that we have two copies of chromosome number one, two copies of chromosome number two and so on. A lot is now understood about the genetic basis for Alzheimer's disease and we know for instance that abnormalities of genes on chromosomes one, fourteen and twenty-one affect the inheritance of Alzheimer's disease, and that are often also involved. We are also beginning to gain some insight into how these abnormalities cause the disease, which, in turn, may lead to treatments that in the future could prevent the disease from progressing.

Other genetic factors also influence whether or not a person may develop Alzheimer's disease. This involves genes that do not cause the disease but increase the likelihood that a person may develop it in the presence of some other contributory factor, or factors. In other words it is rather like the risk of developing lung cancer and smoking. A person may inherit a genetic suscept-ibility or tendency to develop lung cancer but if they don't inhale tobacco smoke lung cancer may never develop, despite the fact that they have the genetic ability for tobacco smoke to cause such a cancer. These are really 'risk factor' genes and a number are being investigated in Alzheimer's disease.

The most prominent of the risk factor genes at the moment is one known as apolipoprotein E. This is also known as ApoE, and it is responsible for making a protein that can exist in three main forms, ApoE2, ApoE3, and ApoE4. We know that ApoE4 confers an increased risk of a person developing Alzheimer's disease. However, it is only a risk factor and does not mean that a person with this gene will necessarily develop Alzheimer's disease and many people with an ApoE4 do not ever develop the symptoms of a dementia, nor does everybody with Alzheimer's disease have ApoE4 gene. Confusing, isn't it?

In summary, the main benefit of knowing about these risk factor genes is that they increase our insight into the ways in which Alzheimer's disease may be caused, but they are of little interest to ordinary people at the moment as they do not reliably indicate who will develop the disease nor do they help much with the diagnosis.

As our understanding of the important role of these risk factor genes increases, they may turn out to be helpful in a number of ways, such as indicating which person may respond better to certain treatments or how their disease may develop in the future. This is the subject of much research at the moment.

To summarize, genes are important in two ways. In a very small number of families where the disease is inherited and manifests itself in earlier life, inheritance of an abnormal gene may cause the person carrying it to develop the disease. There are also other genes, the risk factor genes, all of which are normal but which occur in different forms. In some people some forms of these risk factor genes may increase the likelihood of developing Alzheimer's disease, but only in conjunction with other factors. Possession of a risk factor gene does not necessarily mean that the person possessing this will develop Alzheimer's disease.

Treatments

Knowledge of the biochemical abnormalities in the brain in Alzheimer's disease has at last led to the development of treatment that helps some people. This is mainly based on a knowledge of the lack of the chemical messenger, acetylcholine, that occurs in Alzheimer's disease. There are a number of medicines now available which preserve the decreasing amounts of acetylcholine that are produced in the Alzheimer's disease brain. One called Cognex has been prescribed in the United States for a number of years, and elsewhere, but not in the UK. It has been associated with unpleasant side-effects in some people and newer drugs that work in a similar way are now becoming available. These include Aricept and Exelon, with others in the pipeline. They provide some symptomatic benefit to a little under half of people with mild to moderate dementia caused by Alzheimer's disease, and may slow the progression of symptoms. They are, however, not a cure for the disease. Like all medicines they have some unwanted side-effects of their own, but in most people these do not occur and, if they do, they are relatively short-lived, especially as the dose of medicine is reduced.

Most doctors working in this field believe that these drugs are worthwhile and that everybody with a diagnosis of probable Alzheimer's disease who has mild to moderate symptoms should have the opportunity of a trial of treatment. Unfortunately, in the UK at the time of writing there is considerable variability in the availability of these new medicines as some health authorities do not believe that they offer a significant enough benefit to justify their expense. A three-month trial is usually required to decide whether or not the person for whom the medicine has been prescribed is benefiting sufficiently to warrant longer-term treatment. I hope that by the time this book appears in print this unsatisfactory state of affairs, that is the availability of these new medicines in only some parts of the country, will be a thing of the past.

As well as attempts to try to improve the biochemical changes in the brain in Alzheimer's disease, other strategies are also being developed which we hope will arrest the progression of the disease and perhaps even prevent the formation of the amyloid and the neurofibrillary tangles. There are some promising lines of research underway in this respect and many of us are looking forward to this resulting in the production of new medicines to prevent disease progression rather than just help with the symptoms, which drugs like Aricept and Exelon can do in some people for a year to two at the most.

As is described in a later chapter on research, some other apparently unrelated therapeutic strategies may also be helpful, involving oestrogen, some anti-inflammatory drugs, and also what are known as 'anti-oxidant' substances such as vitamin E. There is preliminary evidence that these and related approaches may affect disease progression, but this needs confirmation with further research.

Tests

Despite our increasing knowledge of the abnormalities that cause Alzheimer's disease we still do not have a single reliable test. Improvement in CT scans is helpful but not sufficiently specific or available to everybody, and there is as yet no simple blood test that will diagnose this condition. This may be a reflection of the fact that Alzheimer's disease is not really a single disease after all, but the final common pathway for a number of different processes. Nevertheless, the search for a diagnostic test goes on and this is further discussed in the chapter on research.

5

Vascular Dementia (VaD)

As has been mentioned already in an earlier chapter, it used to be thought that most, if not all, dementia in older people was a consequence of a disturbance of the blood flow to the brain, in particular a clogging-up of the arteries because of arteriosclerosis. This eventually proved to be untrue, and dementia associated with a disturbance of the blood supply to the brain was thought for many years to be almost entirely the result of multiple small strokes, often called multiple infarct dementia (MID). The term infarct refers to death of tissue because of an absence of blood flow. For many years the concept of MID was considered to be the second most common cause of dementia, and many people are still under this impression. In all fairness, some people with a vascular cause for their dementia do indeed have multiple small infarcts or strokes which are probably causing the patient's difficulties. In general, however, we now know that there are a lot of different ways in which disturbance of the blood supply to the brain can cause dementia, and they are grouped together under the term vascular dementia (VaD). In many people the main problem is associated with damage to very small blood vessels and the effect this has on the white matter within the brain. In some people a single large stroke can cause dementia, though this is not common, and in others a fluctuation in the blood flow may also play a part.

Typically a stroke causes paralysis of the limbs and the face on one side of the body, but there are many areas of the brain where a stroke can affect the intellect without leaving any tell-tale outward signs in the rest of the body. In some cases, however, there is a mixture resulting in both physical abnormalities and intellectual difficulties.

Interestingly, although Dr Alzheimer is usually associated with the condition that now bears his name, he also worked in the field of vascular dementia. Whilst working in an asylum in Frankfurt he published a short report describing arteriosclerotic changes in the brain and recorded symptoms and signs that are very similar to the picture we see nowadays in some people with vascular dementia. Although he described this in late middle age, most people with vascular dementia are in their seventies and eighties.

Changes in the brain

When MID does occur, small areas of brain tissue, at different times, suddenly lose their blood supply because of a blockage. This may lead to physical changes in other parts of the body, for example paralysis or partial paralysis of the limbs on one side, or of one side of the face. Often, however, there is no outward sign of any brain damage, other than the onset of confusion or memory loss. The severity of the person's symptoms is usually related to the amount of brain tissue that is damaged, and also the sites at which this damage takes place within the brain. In many cases the source of the blockage is outside the brain, with small particles or clots travelling along the arterial system from a site elsewhere, for example the heart or one of the large blood vessels between the heart and the brain. This particle or clot is carried along in the blood flow until it reaches a small blood vessel that it cannot get through, and which it then blocks completely.

In some people the block originates within the small blood vessels themselves because of some form of local damage upon which a new clot forms, or a similar process takes place. One of the features of MID, when it occurs, is that the patient's symptoms often progress in a step-wise manner, with a deterioration in ability each time after a small blockage has been created, sometimes with some improvement in the days that follow, but usually only a partial recovery occurs, if at all.

It used to be thought that at least ten teaspoonfuls – 50ml – of brain tissue had to be killed before a dementia occurred but we now know that this is not the case. A single strategically placed area of infarction (brain tissue death) in a vital part of the brain can cause dementia even if it is only a few ml in size.

In those people who do not have MID, probably the majority of people with a vascular dementia, the most important changes occur in the small blood vessels and can only really be seen under the microscope, although sometimes one can see a particular appearance on the CT scan if the process has been severe enough. Partial or complete blockage of these small blood vessels leads to malfunctioning of brain cells and some of their fibres, and also the death of some of them.

The concept of 'vascular cognitive impairment'

A new concept is increasingly being recognized in relation to vascular dementia. It is called vascular cognitive impairment and is extremely important. Inherent in the term vascular cognitive impairment is the recognition that vascular problems slowly accumulate, and that it is often possible to recognize that this process is going on in a person's brain well before they develop an obvious dementia, caused by the increasing accumulation of subtler levels of decreased intellectual ability. If these are recognized, even though the person who is affected does not have a frank dementia, it may be possible to arrest or slow down the vascular damage, avoiding or delaying the onset of the dementia. This means that if a person complains that their mental abilities are not what they were, and there is evidence that there may be a vascular basis for this, even though they have not developed a dementia, the doctor still has the responsibility to find out why their intellect is waning and to see whether he or she can do anything about it.

Many factors can contribute to vascular damage in the brain. These include abnormalities of heart rhythm, changes in the qualities of the cells in the blood, an increased level of fat in the blood, diabetes, high blood pressure, and many more. A search for these possible contributory causes, and their treatment, will sometimes improve brain function, and at the very least will often slow down progression of the illness. In addition to treating the underlying factors, many people will be prescribed a very low dose of aspirin. This makes some of the cells in the blood less sticky and may help the blood to circulate through the brain more effectively. Some people, of course, are unable to take aspirin and other medicines that act in a similar way are available. We do, however, need more evidence, like that which we have for their efficacy in some forms of heart disease, to show just how effective these measures are in the treatment of vascular brain disease.

Symptoms and signs

Vascular dementia can present in a way that is almost indistinguishable from Alzheimer's disease, and other similar conditions, or can develop in a manner that sets it apart. This makes its diagnosis difficult in many cases and when it occurs alongside another cause of dementia, i.e. is one of two conditions affecting the same individual, diagnosis becomes even more fraught with difficulty.

Alzheimer's disease starts in a fairly characteristic manner in most people, with the early signs being deterioration in short-term memory, followed by language difficulty, failing to recognize objects and people, and difficulty with everyday activities. There is a smooth progression as the disease advances, and no evidence of a sudden start or deterioration. Vascular dementia can mimic this, but in many people the pattern of disease progression is different. The order in which symptoms develop depends upon the order in which different parts of the brain are affected and this does not always happen in the same manner as in Alzheimer's. This is where a detailed neuropsychological assessment by a psychologist can be very helpful. If the pattern of intellectual deficit is not what one would expect for the stage of the dementia were it to be Alzheimer's disease, other diagnostic possibilities have to be considered, and the presence of risk factors for vascular disease may well point to the possibility of a vascular cause for the dementia. In addition, many people with vascular dementia retain insight into their condition until much later in the disorder than happens with some of the other illnesses that cause dementia.

Mrs Brown

Mrs Brown was sixty-eight when her husband took her along to their general practitioner because he was worried about her forgetfulness. It was clear that she had been becoming more and more forgetful and that this had started suddenly, after she had experienced a 'dizzy turn' on Christmas Eve. Although she had never lost consciousness, she had had several more funny turns, after most of which she was a little confused for a day or two. The doctor knew that Mrs Brown suffered from diabetes and needed to take tablets, so he checked the level of sugar in her blood. This was normal and she didn't have any of the other symptoms of high blood sugar. He therefore examined her carefully and discovered that she had a high blood pressure. He treated this with the appropriate medicines.

When he saw her again a month later, Mrs Brown was still very forgetful, had some difficulty with her speech, and needed a little help with dressing. This was only a little better than her condition when he had seen her a month previously.

A further year passed, during which Mrs Brown was seen on several occasions by her doctor, who ensured that her blood sugar level and her high blood pressure were properly treated. During this year she had only had one further dizzy spell, after which she had become a little more confused. Although there was some recovery over the ensuing two or three days, she was a little more muddled than before.

In summary, Mrs Brown had some of the characteristic features of multiple infarct dementia and careful attention to the underlying risks – the blood sugar level and the high blood pressure – had probably slowed down the rate of intellectual deterioration.

Treatment

The reader will already be aware that there is little one can do in most cases to guarantee the return of the intellectual function that has been lost. Treatment measures fall, in broad terms, into two categories. The first of these of course is the treatment of any underlying cause: making sure that high blood pressure is brought down to normal levels and kept there; that the blood sugar level is kept within normal limits if the patient has a diabetic tendency; and the second is that the blood is 'thinned' if there is a danger of small blood clots entering the circulation from the heart or the large arteries.

Since the course of vascular dementia is much more erratic than that of most of the other conditions that cause intellectual decline, and since it depends mainly upon the rate at which vascular damage occurs, and the structures within the brain that are affected, it is more difficult to give guidance to families as to what the future holds. It is important that families should know, however, that whereas most people with an Alzheimer's type dementia eventually die of pneumonia, a significant proportion of vascular dementia sufferers, because of abnormalities in arteries outside the head, die as a result of heart failure or coronary thrombosis.

6

Lewy Body Dementia

Lewy body dementia is named after Dr Lewy, who first described the structures that are found inside some brain cells, and which now bear his name. He was originally called Dr Levy, but the world has anglicized his name. Lewy bodies are well known to many doctors as a globular or spherical structure that is found inside some nerve cells in the brain, especially in Parkinson's disease, where they are present in some of the brain cells lying more deeply within the brain's substance. They are a well-known feature of Parkinson's disease and help to confirm the diagnosis when the brain is viewed under a microscope. That Lewy bodies can also be found in the cerebral cortex – the outer layer of grey matter in the brain – has been known for a while but only really came to the fore about ten years ago when more effective ways of showing their presence became available. It then became clear that dementia associated with Lewy bodies was quite a frequent cause of dementia and although it does not occur as frequently as Alzheimer's disease, it is one of the three most frequently occurring conditions.

Lewy body dementia, however, is not the same as Parkinson's disease in which a dementia is also present. In Parkinson's disease the structures within the brain that are affected lie quite deeply within the brain's substance, and although psychological abnormalities can develop, the symptoms are very different to those in a person with, say, Alzheimer's disease. In Lewy body dementia, although there may be some Lewy bodies in the deeper-lying structures, the majority are in the cerebral cortex and the disease has many features that are similar to Alzheimer's disease, although there are differences. It is probable that there is a spectrum of Lewy body disorders with Lewy body dementia being at one end and Parkinson's disease at the other. In between there are conditions which overlap and which therefore can cause some confusion.

Lewy body dementia shares many features in common with Alzheimer's disease, including the presence of plaques in the brain. The Lewy bodies, however, are usually present in the absence of neurofibrillary tangles. Nevertheless, the similarities between the two conditions have led some doctors, especially in America, to believe that Lewy body dementia is a variant of Alzheimer's disease, and this is hotly debated.

The similarities between Lewy body dementia and Alzheimer's disease include some of the patient's symptoms, the presence of the plaques, and some similarity in the pattern of loss of neurotransmitters, i.e. chemical messengers, acetylcholine being the one most affected, just as it is in Alzheimer's disease.

Symptoms

People with Lewy body dementia may have memory disturbance and difficulty with language, leading to impairment of the ability to reason. They also have some features suggesting malfunction of the frontal lobes of the brain, including difficulty in planning and carrying out simple activities, and difficulty with visuospatial function. Sometimes, however, their memory is surprisingly intact.

The features of the dementia associated with Lewy body disease that particularly suggest that this may be the diagnosis include the presence of hallucinations. These tend to occur earlier in the course of the illness than they do in other types of dementia and are usually experienced in the form of 'well-formed' hallucinations, such as seeing a person or an animal when, in reality, nothing is present. Sometimes the person concerned is aware that this is a hallucination and is often remarkably unperturbed by it.

Another feature that is frequently associated with Lewy body dementia is the manner in which the intellectual ability of the sufferer can fluctuate quite dramatically, even from hour to hour. Sometimes this makes doctors think that a confusional state caused by medicines or infection is present, but this can usually be excluded quite quickly. No one knows why there is such a dramatic fluctuation in some people with this disease.

As one might expect, another feature of Lewy body dementia is the presence of symptoms and signs reminiscent of Parkinson's disease in some sufferers. Although this can also occur in other causes of dementia, this type of symptom usually occurs at a later stage. Parkinsonian symptoms can include slowness of movement and thought, stiffness in the arms and legs, a change in posture to one that is more stooped, and a shuffling gait.

Another feature that frequently occurs in people with Lewy body dementia is a tendency to fall for no obvious reason. This happens, of course, to many older people and is not such a good pointer to the presence of the disease as some of the other features mentioned above but, nevertheless, it indicates that Lewy body dementia should be considered as a possibility in a person with dementia who has also been falling.

Diagnosis

As with some of the other conditions, for example Alzheimer's disease and vascular dementia, there is no simple diagnostic test to confirm the presence of Lewy body dementia. It is the pattern of the patient's illness and the way in which it progresses that is most helpful. The only sure way of making the diagnosis is an autopsy examination of the brain after the sufferer has died.

A number of different synonyms have been adopted to describe this condition, or similar illnesses, and these include senile dementia of Lewy body type, Lewy body disease, dementia associated with Lewy bodies, cortical Lewy body disease, and the Lewy body variant of Alzheimer's disease. This can be confusing but at a practical level probably does not matter very much for most patients.

Treatment

As is the case for Alzheimer's disease, Lewy body dementia is presently incurable and eventually death intervenes, often through an intercurrent illness such as pneumonia affecting a body weakened by the relentless progression of the underlying condition. There is a suggestion that people with Lewy body dementia do not survive quite as long as people with Alzheimer's disease but this is very variable.

Many of the support strategies that have been developed to help improve the quality of life of people with Alzheimer's disease, and also that of their carers, are equally applicable to the support required by sufferers of Lewy body dementia, and also their families. There are, however, a number of important points to bear in mind in relation to treatment with drugs.

The first of these points concerns the chemical messenger system in the brain. As already mentioned there is a similar loss of the chemical messenger, acetylcholine, that is found in the Alzheimer's disease brain. In some people with Lewy body dementia this loss is greater than it usually is in most people with Alzheimer's disease. This means of course that the same approach that is used in Alzheimer's disease to preserve the decreasing amounts of acetylcholine available may be helpful in Lewy body dementia. Indeed we know that some people with this condition have been helped by some of the new drugs for Alzheimer's disease as they were unwittingly included in studies designed to evaluate such treatments. When some of these people died and their brains were examined at autopsy, to everyone's surprise it was discovered that a small proportion had Lewy body dementia rather than Alzheimer's disease, and the records from the trial showed that they had improved during the course of their treatment. Cognex, Aricept and Exelon all work by preventing the destruction of the small amounts of acetylcholine being produced, and may well prove useful in Lewy body dementia. At the present time trials of this approach are underway and by the time this book is published we should have a better idea as to whether they offer real hope to the sufferer of a Lewy body dementia.

If a person with a Lewy body dementia develops Parkinson's disease-type symptoms, especially those affecting movement, for example limb stiffness, they may well respond, at least partly, to the drugs that are usually prescribed for Parkinson's disease, especially those containing a substance known as Levodopa. Some of the older anti-Parkinsonian drugs may, however, make their dementia worse and this has to be borne in mind when choosing an appropriate treatment. Treatments in this category are unlikely to improve mental ability – their main benefit being on the movement side, although there have been some claims for efficacy when certain anti-Parkinsonian drugs have been tried in people with dementia.

People with Lewy body dementia often experience hallucinations early in the course of their illness, as described earlier. In addition, they may also suffer other psychiatric disturbances which require treatment. Where this is necessary a group of medicines called neuroleptics are frequently used, for example thioridazine and haloperidol. These should be avoided where at all possible in people with Lewy body dementia and only used under very careful supervision if their prescription is essential. People with Lewy body dementia are particularly sensitive to these medicines, which can cause them harm.

Conclusions

Although Lewy body dementia has only relatively recently been recognized, we already know a lot about it and have considerable understanding of what is happening within the brain when it is affected by this disease. Its similarity with Alzheimer's disease may make it easier for us to develop therapeutic strategies, whilst its different features help us to distinguish it from Alzheimer's disease.

7

Research into Alzheimer's Disease

Our knowledge of Alzheimer's disease is advancing rapidly and since I was preparing the first edition of this book nearly ten years ago, our knowledge has increased enormously. Research in the last ten years has enabled us to both develop and evaluate new treatments for the symptoms of Alzheimer's disease and to understand the basic underlying processes of Alzheimer's disease such that we now have therapeutic strategies emerging that may slow down the disease or prevent it from progressing, and at the same time our understanding of some of the triggers that set off Alzheimer's disease is beginning to make sense. This chapter will concentrate on some of the important additions to knowledge that have led to the development of the treatments that are now available, future therapeutic strategies, and will also discuss the ongoing search for a diagnostic test.

The disease's different patterns

Most doctors, and others working with them in a professional capacity, have a reasonably clear idea about the course of Alzheimer's disease and use this information when making a diagnosis or advising a family about the future. There is nevertheless a considerable degree of variability in the way in which Alzheimer's disease alters a person's physical and psychological character. Sometimes these differences relate to the timing of the onset of symptoms; sometimes they are qualitative differences. There-fore, when a doctor tries to help a family to plan ahead, his or her advice is based on knowledge of the 'average patient' with this condition. A more accurate picture can only be obtained if the medical adviser is able to study a sufferer over a period of time, getting to know that person as an individual and the particular characteristics of his or her condition. Even then it can be very difficult to forecast the future.

It has been found for instance that there is a very small sub-group of people, apparently with Alzheimer's disease, in whom the condition is relatively benign. In these subjects the disease either progresses very slowly or may even seem to cease progression beyond a certain stage.

This variability has led doctors to study the *clinical presentation*, or pattern, of the complex symptoms and signs in the hope that by identifying sub-groups of these symptoms we may be better able to predict the course of dementias in a variety of patients displaying different symptoms. There is also the possibility that Alzheimer's disease may not be a single condition, and that studying different patterns of illness may help sort out different underlying causes. The different patterns of disease presentation may indicate people whose illness could respond to different treatment strategies, and now that we have the earliest drugs for treating Alzheimer's disease, this is being explored. It is also probable that the variability of the course of the illness is a reflection of the multifactorial aetiology, that is the many different underlying contributory factors, some genetic and some environ-mental. This is beginning to indicate to many of us that Alz-heimer's disease could either be considered to be an umbrella term to include a number of different conditions or, alternatively, could be seen as a single disease but with many different causes. In either case, understanding the reason for the differences may help us to tailor treatment, and one day even prevention, more effectively to an individual person's disease process.

Similarity with other conditions

Another reason for studying in detail the way in which the disease affects people is that it may be possible to develop better ways, both of differentiating Alzheimer's disease from other illnesses, particularly vascular dementia and Lewy body dementia, and also of recognizing when one of these and Alzheimer's disease co-exist. Even though it is possible to differentiate these conditions with quite a high degree of accuracy, a confident diagnosis is still much more difficult than with many other problems.

Although Alzheimer's disease is usually regarded as a single condition, there is sufficient similarity of symptoms and signs with other conditions to confuse even the most experienced doctor on occasions. In the present state of knowledge, accuracy in making this diagnosis is of the order of 80–90 per cent. This may well surprise many readers as it means the diagnosis may be wrong for as many as one person in five. This is of particular importance for the trial of new treatments; if it is known that there is a one in five chance of incorrectly including people without Alzheimer's disease in a study of a new medicine, this means that the treatment must be expected not to work in at least one fifth of cases. This has to be taken into consideration when assessing the results of clinical trials of these new medicines.

Parkinsonian stiffness

Among the different groups of people with Alzheimer's disease that stand out are those who develop movement abnormalities. Parkinson's disease is well known because it causes a clearly visible tremor or trembling of the hand or foot and eventually often the whole arm or leg. It also has many other symptoms, including a particular form of stiffness in the limbs. Some people with Alzheimer's disease can also develop this type of stiffness and it is now known that when this occurs, it often indicates that the underlying disease process is going to be more rapid than for those sufferers who do not have this problem.

However, many people with Alzheimer's have this type of stiffness not because of the disease, but because of some of the medicines that are often given to control more disturbed behaviour. It should be possible for a doctor to differentiate between the drug-induced stiffness and that caused by Alzheimer's disease.

Most people who appear to have Alzheimer's disease but who also have the type of stiffness that is characteristic of Parkinson's disease will, as already mentioned, probably be suffering with a Lewy body dementia. However, both Alzheimer's disease and Parkinson's disease can occasionally occur together in the same person, but this is less common. The intriguing overlap between the two diseases has led to much speculation and some research centres are studying in great detail people who have symptoms and signs of both conditions in the hope that this will give us greater insight into both these illnesses.

This may prove to be a particularly important area of research as there are some similarities in the changes in the brain, both structural and biochemical, in the two conditions. Unravelling these may lead to better treatment strategies and perhaps even to an understanding of the cause of degenerative diseases of the brain.

Dividing people into different sub-groups in this way has been challenged by some researchers, who do not feel that we have, as yet, enough knowledge to undertake this task reliably. Nevertheless many of us working in this field believe strongly that sub-groups do exist – but that they can sometimes only be identified by carefully following up a sufferer over a period of time – and that this knowledge can be used to help families plan for the future with a greater degree of certainty than would otherwise be possible.

Genetic research

This is one of the areas where greatest strides have been made in the last ten years, especially during the last five. As well as knowing which abnormal genes can cause Alzheimer's disease in a small number of families in which they are present, we are aware of a number of genes that increase the risk of developing this condition, as already mentioned in earlier chapters.

One of the most important and exciting aspects of our new knowledge about genes and Alzheimer's disease is its potential contribution to our understanding of the disease processes. The genes control the formation of proteins within the cells in our body, and if an abnormal protein, or a different variety of a normal protein, is being formed and this leads to the development of Alzheimer's disease or an increased likelihood of developing it, knowledge of the changes in the protein structure may give us insight into what is actually happening within the brain cells themselves. This may allow us to develop treatments that correct the adverse effect that these different proteins have upon the biochemistry at a cellular level, and may slow it down or prevent the disease from progressing.

Most of the genetic research has concentrated on understanding the formation and harmful effect of the abnormal protein called amyloid that is laid down in the brain in Alzheimer's disease, but we are increasingly understanding the abnormal processes that lead to the formation of the neurofibrillary tangles that are formed inside the brain cells. It may be that modification of both these abnormal processes will be important in developing the ultimate treatment, but it is possible that the amyloid changes affect the brain cells and somehow or other disrupt their biochemistry, leading to the formation of neurofibrillary tangles. If that is the case then preventing the formation of neurofibrillary tangles may be the final common pathway through which a number of different disease processes work.

Vascular changes and Alzheimer's disease

As already described, vascular dementia is thought to be a separate entity to Alzheimer's disease although the two can occur together. We have, however, known for a long time that the abnormal protein, amyloid, that is deposited within the brain tissue itself can also be found in the walls of some of the small blood vessels in the brain. In some related, but different conditions, the amount of amyloid produced is so great that it causes an illness in its own right that is different to Alzheimer's disease, and is associated with a greater tendency to brain haemorrhage. Although such haemorrhages are not a feature of Alzheimer's disease, the association between amyloid and small blood vessels has always led to the suspicion that there might be a vascular component to Alzheimer's disease. This is an intriguing area that is the subject of much research at the present time and although these mechanisms are uncertain, it does seem as if there may be a relationship between blood vessel changes, particularly in the smaller vessels, and the development of Alzheimer's disease. Whether this is part of the Alzheimer's disease process itself or a contributory factor is, as yet, uncertain. Nevertheless, it is an important issue, that we should have a better understanding of in a few years' time.

Factors affecting disease progression

There have been a number of studies trying to find any hint of risk factors that may affect the development of Alzheimer's disease. Some studies have indicated that a significant head injury may increase, but only in some people, the chance of developing Alzheimer's disease. Numerous studies have investigated a whole host of possible underlying factors, and three in particular have come to the fore in a manner that has indicated that they may have therapeutic potential. These have already been mentioned briefly in an earlier chapter in the context of treatments, but it is only fair to refer to them again here as this knowledge is a result of research undertaken in the last ten years. I am of course referring to the apparent protection afforded to people who may be going to develop Alzheimer's disease by oestrogen replacement treatment in women, the use of anti-inflammatory drugs, and the potential role of some vitamins and similar compounds that stop cellular damage caused by a harmful form of oxygen. These all exemplify the two-stage research process that is involved when looking for leads by studying patients and normal people in the community. An inference from basic science research or a hunch leads the investigators to inquire as to whether a particular process may be protective, or the reverse, and a large cohort of people in the community is then studied over a period of time to investigate this. If the outcome is positive this shows that there is an association between what is being studied in Alzheimer's disease but does not prove that it is causal. The next step is to try to influence the progress of Alzheimer's disease by developing a strategy based upon the findings of the community study, for example treating women with oestrogen who are at risk of developing Alzheimer's disease, or prescribing anti-inflammatory drugs, to see whether or not these interventions have any impact upon the disease itself. If the outcome of these approaches is positive, this helps to prove the original hypothesis and leads to the development of a treatment approach that may be complementary to the use of other medicines. We are now awaiting the outcome of research designed to show whether these approaches are really helpful in preventing or delaying the symptoms of Alzheimer's disease.

Development of diagnostic tests

Brain scanning

In recent years there have been many exciting developments in scanning techniques. It is now possible to have all sorts of brain scan and there have been great hopes that this new high-technology approach to studying diseases of the brain might lead to greater diagnostic accuracy. Some of these new techniques, for example the CT scan – also called a CAT scan – provide very detailed information about any structural changes within the brain, producing pictures that look like X-rays.

The standard X-ray picture consists of a single X-ray plate on which are depicted all the structures that the X-rays have passed through, so that in a chest X-ray the heart, the lungs, the ribs, the skin, and the other structures within the chest are all superimposed one upon the other. CT scanning allows the radiologist to examine pictures of an organ bit by bit, providing much greater detail. Another and newer type of scanning called MRI (*magnetic resonance imaging*) can do this even more effectively. These new scanning techniques have proved of great value in diagnosing many conditions such as strokes, tumours, and multiple sclerosis, and evidence is beginning to emerge that they may be helpful in diagnosing Alzheimer's disease. On the one hand brain scans will indicate whether there is an obvious alternative cause for a person's dementia, on the other it is beginning to become apparent that specialized scanning techniques can show the damage caused to certain parts of the brain that particularly occurs in Alzheimer's disease. Although this is not completely diagnostic, it looks as if it may be a great step forward, but will probably be of limited application in the day-to-day clinical situation, as the scanning technology required is only available to a somewhat limited extent and it would not be possible to scan everyone who appeared to have a dementia that may be caused by Alzheimer's disease.

PET scanning

As well as scanning techniques that examine the structure of the brain and the changes within it, there are also those that measure functional changes, such as the way in which the blood passes through the brain or the manner in which the brain cells use up some of the brain chemicals. One such approach is called PET scanning (*positron emission tomography*). This has revealed particular patterns of abnormality in the way in which the Alzheimer brain uses glucose, for example. One interesting finding, however, is the fact that the impairment of glucose metabolism in the cerebral cortex varies between individuals with Alzheimer's disease, and that this difference appears to reflect the way in which the disease affects the sufferer – that is, which symptoms and signs he or she has developed.

PET scanning is extremely complicated and requires access to radioactive materials, albeit in minute quantities, that are difficult to make and use. It is therefore only available in a few centres.

SPECT scanning

There is a similar and more readily available technique to PET scanning. This is called SPECT and is available in most major hospital centres but the demands upon the resources are such that it is usually only employed to help with the diagnosis in a difficult case. SPECT scanning is usually employed to show the pattern of blood flow through the brain, and different conditions that cause dementia often show different patterns, but there is a degree of overlap such that even this type of scan is not diagnostic. Nevertheless it is another useful piece of clinical information that helps to improve the accuracy of our diagnostic ability.

Monitoring the CSF

Many of the diseases that afflict mankind can be diagnosed with relative ease by examining the blood for abnormal changes or looking for specific diagnostic indicators in other body fluids, for example the urine and, particularly for diseases that affect the nervous system, the cerebrospinal fluid (CSF). There are currently many studies seeking 'peripheral' markers of the presence and severity of Alzheimer's disease. If identified, not only might they help with diagnosis, but they might also assist in monitoring the effectiveness of treatment when this becomes available.

Some of the earliest attempts at isolating diagnostic markers involved examining the CSF for changes in its biochemistry that would reflect the biochemical abnormalities that we know occur in the brain. Although there have been some reports of differences between people with Alzheimer's disease and normal people of the same age without any intellectual deficit, there has been too much overlap between the two groups to enable the biochemical differences in question to indicate reliably the presence or absence of the disease. Similar attempts have been made to examine the changes in the blood and again the results have been disappointing.

More recently, and in many ways more hopefully, researchers have been trying to identify changes in the CSF and the blood that relate not to the biochemical changes within the brain, but to the structural abnormalities that develop in Alzheimer's disease. Attempts are in hand to try and make the diagnosis by proving that the blood or CSF contains substances which indicate that the brain, in its turn, contains more senile plaques or neurofibrillary tangles than it should. At the time of writing this seems a much more logical approach and several tests have arrived at the point of clinical trial. It will probably be a year or two, however, before we know whether they are going to live up to our expectations.

The electroencephalograph

There have of course been many other approaches to developing diagnostic tests for Alzheimer's disease. One of these involves measuring the brain's electrical activity, and the way in which the pattern of different brain waves is affected by underlying abnormalities.

Most people are familiar with the ECG (electro-cardiograph), which is a technique used to measure the electrical activity of the heart and is very useful in diagnosing many cardiac conditions. The equivalent for the the brain is known as an EEG (electroencephalograph), and is a lot more complicated. It certainly does appear as if there are some changes in the brain waves in people with Alzheimer's disease but again they haven't been found to be sufficiently specific to form the basis of a reliable test. Further refinement of the measurement of these very complicated patterns of brain electrical activity and the way in which they alter with the disease may, however, one day prove helpful.

It is essential that reliable diagnostic indicators for Alzheimer's disease are developed, for without them clinical trials of the newer and more hopeful therapeutic strategies will be difficult to interpret, and counselling of relatives of sufferers will continue to be hampered.

Research into structural changes

Inside the brain

Some of the earliest research into Alzheimer's disease involved examining the structural abnormalities that occurred in the brain, and which were visible through a microscope. As more powerful equipment such as the electron microscope became available, the more detailed structural changes within the cells themselves came under scrutiny. Our research into the structural abnormalities has now proceeded even as far as examining the molecular structure of neurofibrillary tangles and some of the components of the senile plaques. In addition to suggesting new treatment strategies, this approach has also increased our understanding of some of the basic disease mechanisms.

Outside the brain

As well as finding abnormalities in the nerve cells themselves and also their fibres, we have discovered that there are changes, including the formation of neurofibrillary tangles, in at least one structure outside the brain itself. The nerve fibres that are associated with our sense of smell pass from the nose through small holes in the skull to a pair of structures about the size of a grain of wheat, one on each side. These are known as the *olfactory bulbs* and are connected to the brain. Those parts of the brain that are important for appreciating and distinguishing between different smells are very heavily afflicted with neurofibrillary tangles, and we now know that the olfactory bulbs are similarly affected. Although this finding may well turn out to be a red herring, it could indicate one route of entry into the brain of a toxic substance or infectious agent such as a virus. It would be relatively easy for some viruses that live in the nose to pass into the brain along this pathway and then to spread to different parts of the brain.

The link with Down's syndrome

People with Down's syndrome are now living much longer than they used to and with this has come the realization that most, and possibly all if they survive long enough, will develop a condition that is the same as or very similar to Alzheimer's disease. The brain of a person with Down's syndrome shows at a relatively early age the formation of the plaques and tangles that are so much part of the picture of Alzheimer's disease. In addition to the structural changes there are also similar biochemical abnormalities. Whether or not older people with Down's syndrome are particularly likely to develop dementia is, however, a matter of contention, as with so many other aspects of Alzheimer's disease. In one study, less than half of the group of Down's syndrome sufferers over the age of fifty demonstrated significant intellectual decline; in others, psychological impairments characteristic of Alzheimer's have been found in the majority if not all.

Part of the problem lies in the fact that we don't have adequate tests to measure dementia in people who have a pre-existing intellectual problem. The existing tests on previously normal people are difficult enough to interpret, so results for people with Down's syndrome can be very misleading. This is particularly true if all the Down's syndrome subjects are studied only once and a judgement made as to whether, at say the age of fifty, they are suffering from a dementia-like illness. The best way of deciding whether or not dementia is an inevitable accompaniment to increasing age in Down's syndrome is to undertake a longitudinal study. This means regular assessment over a period of time, providing an opportunity to compare change in intellectual ability over a number of years. Further research of this type is needed, but if it is confirmed that subjects with Down's syndrome can exhibit the abnormal changes in the brain that occur in Alzheimer's disease, yet do not all develop dementia or significant intellectual decline, then this would have important implications for the significance of the presence of senile plaques and neurofibrillary tangles, etc., in the diagnosis of Alzheimer's disease.

The presence of plaques and tangles in the brains of people with Down's syndrome stimulated examination of *chromosome 21*. As already described, the chromosomes are the structures on which all genes lie, and in Down's syndrome there is extra chromosome 21 material. At one time it was postulated that people with Alzheimer's disease also had extra chromosome 21 material. It was therefore possible to conjecture that an excess of genetic material on chromosome 21 may cause the abnormalities in the brain in both Alzheimer's disease and Down's syndrome. This view appeared particularly attractive when it was discovered that the gene responsible for the formation of amyloid, the substance in the centre of the senile plaque, was also on chromosome 21. It seemed as if at least part of the cause of Alzheimer's disease had been found. We now know that it is not as simple as this; although chromosome 21 is implicated in the development of the senile plaque protein, it seems that the earlier hypothesis that this particular gene was the Alzheimer gene is unlikely to be true in most people, and there is no evidence that Alzheimer's disease sufferers have extra chromosome 21 material.

Aluminium and mercury

It is possible that the brain of some sufferers with Alzheimer's disease contains an unusual quantity of aluminium. It now also seems fairly clear that the aluminium is especially concentrated in those structures that are most affected in Alzheimer's disease and that it is found in association with the senile plaques and the neurofibrillary tangles. This of course has led to considerable speculation that aluminium could be the cause of, or a contributory factor to, the development of this type of dementia in at least some sufferers, if not most. Despite this, there is still considerable uncertainty, as some researchers believe that the apparent accumulation of aluminium is really an artifact of the way in which the brain is processed once it is removed from the body of an Alzheimer's disease sufferer who has died. In other words the accumulation of the aluminium is the result of the way in which the brain is processed rather than something that was present within it whilst the sufferer was alive.

The aluminium theory was further strengthened by the results of experiments on animals that have shown neurofibrillary-tangle-like structures developing in brain cells exposed to large quantities of aluminium. Further, people with kidney failure who have to undergo renal dialysis run the risk of developing a confusional state if the dialysis procedure allows too much aluminium to enter their body. Although this is now rigorously controlled, in earlier days before the relationship between aluminium and brain damage in kidney patients was established, some people with kidney failure died of a condition known as *dialysis encephalopathy*. Excess levels of aluminium were implicated in this process.

Although this all makes for a good *prima facie* case for aluminium as a potential cause of Alzheimer's disease, one has to remember that aluminium might be accumulating in the brain as a result of the condition rather than as an agent which is causing it. It is possible that damaged tissue may accumulate aluminium in greater quantities than undamaged tissue. Most people working in this field believe that aluminium accumulates passively as a consequence of ageing or damage to brain cells, and maybe also as a consequence of the processing of the brain at autopsy. Moreover, accumulation of aluminium is known to occur in other brain disorders, in which the characteristic changes of Alzheimer's disease do not occur. The people dying of dialysis encephalopathy did not develop the same changes in the brain as are found in Alzheimer's disease, or if they did, to only a very minor and possibly insignificant extent. In addition, aluminium does not accumulate in all places where plaques and tangles occur and in at least one study it was found not to have accumulated in that part of the brain that is usually most severely affected by the abnormal changes. If aluminium really were important, one would have expected the highest levels in this area – the hippocampus.

A lot of prominence has been given to the level of aluminium in drinking water. Aluminium is added to the water supply as part of the purification process and in many parts of the country water has a naturally high level of aluminium dissolved in it.

Although a recent study claims that Alzheimer's disease appeared to be more common in parts of the country with higher than average levels of aluminium in the water, even this evidence is not strong enough to implicate aluminium as the cause of Alzheimer's disease.

The study is a difficult one to interpret for a number of reasons: although in general it was reported that there were more cases of Alzheimer's disease in areas where the water was high in aluminium, some areas with the highest levels were not associated with the greatest number of cases. Besides, we take in a lot more aluminium with our food than in our drinking water. The latter is responsible for only a small proportion of the 5–6mg of aluminium that most adults ingest each day.

If aluminium is one day shown to be an important contributory factor and the scepticism of many of us shown to be inappropriate, it will prove very difficult to minimize our intake of the substance. Aluminium is one of the most common elements in the earth's crust and is present all around us. Not only does it occur in our water and naturally in our food, it is a common component of some food additives. It is present in cosmetics and talcum powder and in the dust that we breathe.

In any case the link, if one exists, between aluminium and Alzheimer's disease is unlikely to be a simple matter of cause and effect. Two people can live side by side for sixty years, having got married in their late teens or early twenties, consuming a very similar amount of aluminium throughout their life. Only one of them develops Alzheimer's disease and their neighbours, who probably have a not dissimilar lifestyle, are also spared. Why this selectivity? It is possible that some subjects with Alzheimer's disease inherit a tendency to be particularly sensitive to aluminium or process it within their nervous systems in an abnormal manner. Although this possibility does exist, there is as yet no firm evidence in its favour.

Finally, an alternative and totally speculative hypothesis involves the suggestion that the aluminium that we consume during our adult lives is irrelevant and that if this element plays any part at all in causing Alzheimer's disease, it is aluminium intake in early life, perhaps even before birth, that is important, causing damage to nerve cells in the brain which does not become apparent until much later in life. There is, however, no evidence at all at the moment to support this possibility and I only mention it for the sake of interest. In general I think that most people working in this field would probably agree that aluminium is unlikely to be a major factor in the development of Alzheimer's disease, but that it is not possible to state with complete certainty that it has no role to play in some individuals. At the time of writing, however, the evidence is inadequate to suggest throwing out those aluminium cooking pots and pans!

Mercury is known to have a toxic effect on the brain and the rest of the nervous system. Nevertheless, there has been no consistent evidence that mercury levels in the brain are related to the development of Alzheimer's disease. This possibility was, however, a source of concern as mercury is one of the constituents of some of the older types of dental amalgam – tooth fillings used by dentists. It does not seem as if people with more fillings are more likely to develop dementia of any sort and this seems to be a theoretical rather than a practical worry.

Participating in research

There are no adequate animal models of Alzheimer's disease and therefore most of the research findings discussed in this chapter are based upon research that has taken place either involving brain tissue donations from affected and normal individuals, the latter for comparative purposes, or from the study of sufferers while they are alive. This is beginning to change a little, as the ability to insert human disease genes into laboratory animals, i.e. transgenic animals, has resulted in an improved ability to understand what happens in the brain when brain cells are affected by abnormal genes. Nevertheless, Alzheimer's disease is such a complex process that it is unlikely that we will ever be able to understand all we need to as a result of these transgenic animal experiments. I am also aware that many readers of this book may believe that such animal experiments are unethical and inappropriate, but this is not the place to discuss this issue further. Most of these experiments are being undertaken in the United States and other parts of Europe, and we will have to await their outcome. In the meantime, I and many others believe that we have much to learn by studying the disease processes in our patients, and also by studying normal people so that we can draw comparisons.

There are many different ways in which a person with dementia can contribute to research, ranging from providing blood samples, to undergoing new types of scanning, to in-depth studies of what is happening within their memory functions. In addition all the new medicines have to be evaluated carefully to establish that they are effective and safe.

We don't like to include people with dementia in any form of research unless we feel they have given their consent. This can be very difficult because the more severe the dementia the more limited the person's understanding, but all researchers have to go to great lengths to try and ensure that the subjects in their research are not unwilling, and no pressure must ever be put upon them, or their carers. We also stress that refusal to take part in a research project will in no way affect the nature or level of care that they will receive in the future. Research is also, in nearly every case, undertaken on an 'anonymous' basis, and no individual is named.

As well as trying to obtain the consent of the person who has the dementia, most researchers also involve the carer or next of kin, and if they indicate that they are unwilling for the research to take place, especially if it is because they feel that the person with Alzheimer's disease has not really given their consent, or would not have liked to take part, then this is a decision that would be respected.

Not all research is going to help the person who takes part in it, and many studies are more likely to help future generations of Alzheimer's disease sufferers. This of course raises an ethical issue when a person is unable to give informed consent. It would be unusual for a person with dementia to be included in a study that did not have the opportunity of helping them as an individual unless they were able to give informed consent.

As well as involving the person with dementia and their relatives or carers, all research has to be passed by an Ethics Committee consisting of a panel of medical people balanced by lay people and other professionals. They are there to safeguard the individual rights of the person with dementia, and will not allow a study to be undertaken unless they believe that the procedures involved are ethically acceptable and that the research will eventually lead to some benefit to people suffering with the disease that is being studied.

Research therefore sometimes provides an opportunity for the person participating to obtain some benefit, will usually provide knowledge that will help in the future, even if the person participating does not benefit, and will often enable relatives and carers to make a contribution if they are given the opportunity of deciding whether or not to participate as a normal or 'control' subject for comparative purposes.

Donating brain tissue after death is another means of supporting research. This does not usually delay the funeral arrangements or disfigure the person who has died. Arrangements are best made in advance, in anticipation of helping research in this way, so that there is not a last-minute panic looking for a suitable research centre at a time of sadness to all involved. The Alzheimer's Disease Society has some very helpful information sheets about volunteering for research and also making brain tissue donations. These are well worth reading and will answer most people's questions.

In conclusion

Enormous strides have been made in the last ten to fifteen years in our understanding of the changes in the brain, and outside it, in Alzheimer's disease and some of the other dementias. This information has been very helpful in the search for underlying causes and in the attempts to develop more effective treatments. I firmly believe that we are presently at the most important and exciting phase of the drive to conquer Alzheimer's disease. We should look forward to the future with confidence and hope.

8

The Services Available and How to Use Them

This chapter details the medical, social and voluntary services that are, or should be, available to help families to care for a person with dementia in their own home for as long as possible. Everyone involved in looking after a relative or friend with dementia at home, or who is employed to care for people with dementia, should have a clear idea of what support is available, what and for whom it can reasonably be expected to provide, and how to gain access to it when required. Many people will discover that some of the services described in this chapter are not available in their own area. Sometimes this is because of a lack of resources, but sometimes it results from flexibility in the health and social services planning for the problems of a particular area. Local circumstances tend to dictate the level of provision of services.

The general practitioner

The general practitioner is usually the key person involved in organizing the care for anybody living at home with a chronic degenerative condition. It is essential that both patient and carers have confidence in and get on with their family doctor. Unfortunately there are always going to be some people who feel that the relationship with their general practitioner is unsatisfactory. This is, however, often as much the fault of the patient and the patient's family as it is of the doctor.

Many patients visit their doctor and for a host of reasons fail to get across why they have really made the appointment. It is easy to describe a simple physical problem that can be demonstrated such as a rash or a swollen joint, but often much more difficult to describe adequately less tangible conditions, particularly those associated with stress. Before visiting your doctor therefore it is important to get quite clear in your own mind what the problem really is and how it has affected your day-to-day life. This means, whether the problem is affecting you or someone else, deciding in your own mind what is really wrong. You also need to have an idea beforehand of what sort of action you hope the doctor will take. If you are worried about forgetting things, jot down a few points on a piece of paper, more in the form of notes to jog your own memory rather than as a lengthy account for the doctor to read.

If you wish to tell the doctor that you are worried about an elderly relative's mental condition, rather than just saying that the person in question is becoming more forgetful, be prepared to describe what is happening and how seriously you regard the problem. Have examples ready of how the forgetfulness or muddled thinking is having an important impact on the life of the person concerned and those around them. If you want a careful analysis made of the forgetfulness or confusion, make sure that the doctor is aware that you want a proper assessment of whether the condition is the result of an early form of dementia. You must also be ready to tell him that if it is dementia, you want the underlying cause diagnosed, just in case it is one of the treatable conditions. Try not to make it appear as if you are demanding action, but rather let the doctor know that you are concerned and are seeking support and advice.

If, despite this, the matter doesn't appear to be taken seriously, particularly if the doctor hasn't examined his patient and has not requested a second opinion, tell him that you realize that blood and other tests are probably necessary to rule out conditions such as glandular disorders and nutritional deficiencies, and that you would be prepared to go to hospital for a second opinion if he would prefer that. Above all, don't be put off; but at the same time try to handle the situation tactfully if you think your problems are being treated with insufficient care.

It is very important that you listen carefully to what the doctor says. Most people, including myself, feel anxious when seeking medical advice for themselves or their family. This results in a tendency to want to make sure that the doctor has heard all that you wish to say, often in the way in which you want to say it, which may result in your not answering his questions accurately; more importantly you may not take in what he says to you. If at the end of the consultation you are not quite clear about what has been decided, ask your doctor to summarize the action that he is going to take.

There are all sorts of doctors just as there are all sorts of people. If you don't get on with your doctor you must change to somebody else. This often seems an incredibly difficult obstacle to overcome, but it really is very important. If you are looking after somebody with dementia, you are going to need help, increasingly so, over many years. Doctors realize that they won't always relate well to every patient or relative. If you feel you have this type of problem, summon up the courage to discuss it with your doctor and explain the reasons in a friendly and tactful manner. He will probably understand and a discussion of this nature can often lead to a better understanding, making a change unnecessary. An alternative approach is to arrange to see a different member of the practice on a subsequent occasion. One of the benefits of large group practices is that there is a greater likelihood of most people's needs being met by at least one of the partners.

Changing your general practitioner

It can be very difficult to choose a new general practitioner, either because you have moved into a new area or decided to part company with the practice with which you are currently registered. Ask friends and neighbours who their doctor is and where the surgery is located. Ask them how they get on with their doctor and what they see as the strengths and weaknesses of the doctors they know. If possible, try to make contact with other people caring for a person with dementia and see whether their doctor has the qualities that you think are important.

Make a shortlist of practices – there will probably only be three or four at most within easy reach of your home, fewer in rural areas – and visit them. You can tell a lot from the atmosphere that you pick up as you enter the surgery and from the attitude of the reception staff. Make a list of questions to ask, such as are the doctors taking on new patients, are you in their area, how do you register with them, do they have any particular interests, and do they visit the elderly house-bound. Ask if you can make an appointment to talk to one of the doctors before registering with them. The way in which your questions are treated, and more importantly whether they make you feel welcome, should help you to decide if this is the practice with which you wish to register.

The GPs' medical staff

The doctors in a general practice employ many different staff, especially if they are part of a large and busy partnership. Most people will meet one of the receptionists before they meet their doctor. Some receptionists are better than others, but all should take patients' and relatives' problems seriously and treat them with consideration however harassed they may themselves be feeling. They should never be allowed to make diagnoses and they should never fob patients off. Anything they are told should be treated as confidential; strictly speaking there is no reason at all why they should know anything about the problem that has led to the request for a consultation with the doctor.

Of the other medical staff, older people with dementia are most likely to meet the health visitor or one of the nurses in the practice. The latter is particularly responsible for helping to provide nursing care to sufferers in their own home and this will be more important later on in the case of a dementing illness. In many areas the nurses are supported by auxiliary nurses who help with jobs like washing and bathing. Nurses working in general practice are trained to appreciate the needs, physical and emotional, of patients and their relatives, to provide appropriate care, and to summon up other members of the community health team when required. They will also keep the doctors informed about the physical condition of their patients.

The health visitor is someone who has trained and practised as a nurse and also often as a midwife. She receives additional training, especially in prevention of illnesses. In the past health visitors have tended to concentrate on young people and children but with the increasing numbers of older people they are playing an important role with this age group too. A health visitor will be able to give advice and mobilize extra resources if they are needed. Unfortunately, health visitors are in short supply.

As most readers will be aware, the previous government instituted a series of 'over 75' checks, i.e. each practice is expected to assess the health and well-being of the patients registered with them who are aged seventy-five years or over, and this should include an assessment of mental ability. In different practices the assessment will be undertaken by different professional disciplines and it is often a nurse rather than a doctor who makes the assessment. Whoever it is, this may well prove to be an effective initial first step in obtaining help and advice about an elderly relative whose mental powers are waning.

Hospital services

A young person with suspected dementia will probably first be referred to a neurologist. This is a doctor who has been specially trained in the diagnosis and treatment of disorders of the nervous system, including the brain. Neurologists ensure that a thorough physical examination is undertaken, having carefully inquired into the history of the illness, and will arrange appropriate tests, including blood tests and special X-rays. However, after making a diagnosis, many will not be in a position to offer any regular help and will refer the continuing management of the patient back to the general practitioner.

An older person with dementia is more likely to be referred to a geriatrician or a psychiatrist with a special interest in the elderly, sometimes called a psychogeriatrician. Geriatricians are trained in all the disorders that are found more commonly in older people. They will perform a very similar assessment to that provided by the neurologist for younger people, but will also have access to many of the health service resources that are essential for the continuing care and support for people with dementia, and for their relatives and carers.

Hospital beds to provide intermittent relief or holiday admissions are becoming a less frequent resource of the geriatric department and such a facility may have to be sought by asking for advice from a social worker. Most departments of geriatric medicine, however, still have a day hospital. This is not necessarily a facility for providing relief for families, but an environment in which further careful assessment can be undertaken. In most cases there has to be a 'therapeutic' need for a person to attend a day hospital. Day relief is provided elsewhere, for example at day centres run by the statutory and voluntary services.

Although there are no strict rules, elderly people with dementia who require screening are generally referred first to a geriatrician, but after this the care for those who are mobile as well as demented usually falls to the psychogeriatrician. There are good practical reasons for this; for instance, psychiatric day hospitals are more secure and a wandering demented person is less likely to escape and come to harm. On the other hand a demented person who is heavily dependent on physical nursing will more usually need the help of the geriatric service. There are of course many exceptions to this generalization.

Very often psychogeriatricians will visit patients in their own home, and take the opportunity to familiarize themselves with the problems that relatives and other carers are having to manage. In this way they can judge how best the resources that they have available can help. It also allows those looking after a person with dementia to demonstrate the difficulties they are facing and being able to talk about the problem in their home environment is often easier than trying to describe the situation in a busy out-patient clinic.

Once the matters of diagnosis and assessment have been completed, the specialist will plan the future with the family, the general practitioner, and often other members of his team. It is important that everybody knows about this 'package' so that they can see the way ahead. One must also remember that the package has to be regarded flexibly and its provisions may need to be changed as the situation alters.

In some parts of the country there are specialist clinics for people with dementia where a person with dementia isn't just seen in a slot between people with other conditions, but is assessed in an environment in which all patients have similar problems and all staff are specially trained in this area of medicine. The pattern in different memory clinics varies, but in some every patient is seen by a geriatrician, a psychiatrist and a psychologist, and great attention is paid to the problems and needs of the carers. (A psychiatrist is a doctor trained in the problems of mental illness; a psychologist, although not medically qualified, is trained in the skills of behaviour assessment, behaviour treatment, and other related activities; he or she is also able to give valuable advice.) A full appraisal of the medical problems is made, a diagnosis of the underlying disorder is established, and treatment is prescribed for the fortunate few with a remediable underlying condition. The appropriateness of prescribing one of the new medicines for Alzheimer's disease will also be given consideration, even though in many parts of the country it may not be possible to prescribe this as part of NHS treatment. The way ahead is mapped out and the patients and their families seen regularly two or three times a year. The day-to-day management of patients' care is returned to the general practitioner or to the local specialist if they have been referred from another area of the country. The clinic may also have a support group attached to it for the families of people with dementia who live in the district. The number of clinics like this is increasing, and if one is available locally, your general practitioner will probably seek a second opinion from it. One of the major strengths of such clinics is that they often have a representative of both the geriatric and the psychogeriatric service, allowing closer collaboration between the two in dealing with the needs of a particular person.

Attending a hospital clinic

Much of what has been said about the relationship between patients, relatives, and general practitioners is also true in the context of the hospital clinic. There are, however, several practical points that should be borne in mind. Aim to arrive at least ten minutes before the appointment time or, if parking is likely to be difficult, even earlier. If transport has been arranged by the hospital make sure that you are ready a good quarter of an hour before the time that the ambulance or car is due. It is very likely that you will have to wait for some time both before seeing the doctor and while some of the assessment is taking place, although you will be involved in quite a lot of this yourself. It is important therefore to take something to occupy yourself and if possible something that will occupy your relative with dementia. It is also a good idea to make sure you know where the toilets are and, if you have to make use of them, let the nurse in charge of the waiting area know where you are going, and that you won't be long. If you have to leave your relative in the waiting area, make sure that the nurse in charge knows that he or she will be unattended, particularly if wandering is a problem.

If your appointment is near a mealtime, ask whether there is a cafeteria for patients in the hospital or take sandwiches. It is better to do this than risk going without a meal. Make sure that the clothes your relative is wearing are easy to take off as he or she will probably need to be examined fully.

Remember that the staff at the clinic are there to help you. It may well be more difficult to talk to them than it is to your own general practitioner whom you know better and whom you see in relatively familiar surroundings. Even if the doctors, nurses, and others seem hurried, remember that you have come a long way to see them, probably at great inconvenience to yourself and possibly others, and that it is important that you leave the clinic with a clear idea of the present position and what is going to happen next. After all, if you return home and find that one of your most pressing questions hasn't been answered, it won't be as easy to find out the answer as if you had only to repeat a visit to the general practitioner's surgery.

Despite being well organized, many people nevertheless discover when they arrive home that they have forgotten something that was said or have forgotten to mention something. Don't worry about this! There are two courses of action that you can take. One is to make an appointment to see the family doctor and ask him whether he could answer the question for you or find out the answer. The other approach, possibly the better of the two, is to write a letter to the specialist explaining the position and putting the question.

I would like to stress again that although the staff in hospital clinics may well seem more difficult to approach, either because they are less familiar than the local general practitioner or because they seem exceptionally busy, it is important that you take this opportunity of finding out the answers to your questions. Don't be intimidated by them. As long as you ask your questions in a courteous and friendly manner, you will most likely be treated with consideration.

Admission to hospital

If it is necessary for a person with dementia to go into hospital, whether for a short-term admission or, increasingly less likely, for longer-term care, it is very probable that all sorts of worries and fears will spring up in the minds of relatives. Much of this is caused by the unfamiliarity with the hospital routine and the fear of leaving someone who is much loved in a strange environment with strange people for long periods, not knowing what is happening to them while you are away. Hospitals are making great strides to try to overcome these problems but nevertheless an in-patient stay will often be a stressful event.

A new approach to nursing is being introduced into many hospitals whereby one nurse has special responsibility for a small number of patients, getting to know them and their families well. If this is the system in the ward to which your relative is admitted, find out which of the nurses knows your relative best and try to get to know them.

Of the medical staff, the doctor you will see regularly will be the most junior member of the team. He or she will have responsibility for the day-to-day care of your relative, referring to more senior doctors for advice when necessary. The consultant will probably only see his patients once or twice a week, having trained his team to look after their patients in the way that he expects. He is responsible for the major decisions that are made, but will usually take into account the advice and assessment of all the members of his team, not just the other doctors, but also the physiotherapists and occupational therapists where relevant, and especially the nurses, who will know the patient best.

Often the consultant will be guided by a social worker or a health visitor and sometimes other members of the community health team too. He will also be available to give advice on any urgent medical problems that arise. He will probably have patients in many hospital wards, often in more than one hospital, and other medical duties elsewhere. He is therefore the most difficult person to see, but a telephone call to his secretary should make it possible for you to see him if you feel you would like to – and there is no reason why you shouldn't. In practical terms this is often most easily arranged for a time when he is going to be on your relative's ward.

If the admission has been made to allow assessment and investigation of the underlying causes of a dementia, your relative will undergo quite a lot of tests and will probably be examined by more than one person. This can be disturbing to someone who has a limited capacity to understand what is happening to them. The nurses and doctors will be aware of this and will try to help as much as they can. Unfortunately it isn't always possible to avoid distressing a patient in these circumstances, but in general few patients are significantly upset by their experience. It is also unlikely that any permanent distress will be caused as most people, although not all, with dementia will forget the experience relatively soon. It is important that everyone with dementia is thoroughly assessed and if the hospital admission is necessary, this usually won't be for longer than seven to ten days.

If the admission has been arranged to allow you to have some relief, please don't visit every day. This will defeat the whole purpose of the admission and can in fact make the relief period even more stressful than not having any relief at all. It is quite natural to worry about what is happening and to wish to find out. This can easily be achieved by telephoning the ward and asking to speak to the nurse in charge or the nurse who knows your relative best. Before doing this, however, check with the nurses when is the most convenient time to ring and let them know that you intend to. Having been forewarned, they should then make sure that they are aware of what has been happening to your relative and will be in a position to give you some meaningful information.

Intermittent admissions to hospital for respite relief are becoming less frequently available as many health authorities believe this should be a function of social services or the voluntary sector. Hospital intermittent admission is now usually reserved for those few people who cannot be managed elsewhere than in hospital, and can be arranged in two ways. The first of these is a week or two, once or twice a year, to allow hard-pressed relatives or other carers to get away and have a holiday. The other consists of more frequent, but often shorter, periods in hospital to allow families to recharge their batteries. The latter becomes more important when the demands of caring increase as the disease progresses. In the early stages of the illness, holiday or even intermittent care can often be provided somewhere other than a hospital, for example an old people's home. If the stage is reached where nursing care is required, a nursing home or the equivalent is usually best. The person who will be most up to date with the arrangements for intermittent or holiday care will be the general practitioner.

Community psychiatric nurses (CPNs)

These invaluable members of the health care team are often part of the supporting system for families caring for people with dementia and for the many demented elderly people who are living alone at home despite their illness. They are trained psychiatric nurses and many have also trained in general nursing and can therefore appreciate and understand the physical as well as the psychiatric problems. In some areas they are based in a hospital, attached to a psychiatrist's team; in others they are attached to health centres. Sometimes they operate from both. The CPN liaises across all the different services – social services, geriatric service, psychiatric service – and may have to work closely with the general practitioner. Many of them have close links with the voluntary bodies in the locality. They do not carry out physical nursing tasks; these are the province of the nurses attached to your general practice. A CPN will usually be involved after the general practitioner has referred a patient for assessment to a psychiatric clinic or asked a psychogeriatrician to make a visit to the person's home. In some areas, a general practitioner can himself initiate the CPN's involvement.

The CPN has a wealth of experience and knowledge, will be able to give practical advice about coping with routine problems, may be able to arrange attendance at a day hospital or day centre as appropriate, and can alert others if the need arises.

Local authority support (social services)

The local authority has to provide many different services. These range from home helps – often the mainstay of a care network that enables an old person with dementia to continue living alone or a family to carry on coping – to day-care provision.

Among these services is meals-on-wheels, which aims to ensure at least a basic standard of nutrition on several or most days of the week. In many places this will be contracted out to other agencies. Remember, however, that although the meals-on-wheels service may deliver food, many elderly people with dementia don't eat it! Sometimes this is for practical reasons such as ill-fitting dentures, but often it is because of lack of supervision. I can remember visiting one old lady in her mid-eighties, whose dementia had been a problem for three or four years, but who was still living at home. Her general practitioner had asked me to see her because she was losing weight and was becoming more frail. The house smelt awful and when I went into the scullery, a little room behind the kitchen, I discovered 123 of the meals-on-wheels service's foil containers, mostly unopened, none empty; of those which had been sampled, most looked as if no more than a forkful or two of food had been consumed from them.

The local authority also employs social workers, who are highly trained professionals with a wide range of skills and responsibilities. The social worker, unless based in a geriatric or psychogeriatric department, is very unlikely to work only with the elderly, but nevertheless will be very knowledgeable about the provision of local services. He or she will be trained to advise about welfare entitlements, can provide a list of local nursing and residential homes, and liaises with the home help and meals-on-wheels services.

Social services also run day-care centres. Some of these are specifically for the elderly with dementia. As well as providing some welcome daytime relief for carers, they can also provide a stimulating and pleasant environment for the elderly people who attend. Sadly, however, they are unable to cope with more severely demented people and may require those attending to be mobile. Unless they are specifically established for people with dementia, they may not be able to deal with confused people who wander or those who are aggressive or otherwise more difficult to manage socially.

As well as providing day-care, some social services, and also voluntary bodies, provide sitting services, either at night or in the daytime. This enables a hard-pressed carer to escape from the house and have some freedom without having to make arrangements with day centres or day hospitals. More import-antly, a night-sitting service allows the carer the opportunity of getting a full night's sleep. Continually broken rest at night wears one down and can be the final straw for many carers.

You can find the telephone number of your local social services department in the telephone directory under the name of your local authority. They will be able to send you information about the local services that they provide and also about how to apply for an assessment of the person with dementia needs, and if you are a carer, yours also. A telephone call to the Alzheimer's Disease

Society (see Appendix 1) will also pay dividends here. They have some very useful information sheets about community care assessment, welfare benefits, and other matters such as the council tax, since people with dementia and their carers are often eligible for relief on the council tax charge.

Voluntary organizations

Voluntary organizations tend to provide the same sort of facility and support as those social services already mentioned. These voluntary services often come into being because of a lack of provision by the local authority or health service. They usually spring up as a result of the initiative of an enterprising individual who is or was a carer. They range from day centres, sitting services, lunch clubs and drop-in centres for confused elderly people to support groups for the carers. The latter are described in more detail in chapter 13.

As well as those that arise locally, there are also national voluntary organizations. The Alzheimer's Disease Society, whose address and telephone number are given at the end of this book, is the main source of voluntary input, advice, and help for people caring for relatives or others with dementia, whether or not this is the result of Alzheimer's disease. It has an extensive network of branches and support groups, and also carers' contacts across England, Wales and Northern Ireland, and has a sister organization in Scotland. The local office will be able to tell you what they provide in your area and this may include advice and information, support groups, telephone helplines, and sitting services, or even day care. The national office has an enormous wealth of information and guidance, mainly in the form of leaflets, brochures and other publications, which is unrivalled in this field. Other organizations with a more general remit include Age Concern, Counsel and Care, Help the Aged, and many others. You will find their names, addresses, and telephone numbers in Appendix 1. The first port of call for most people requiring advice from the voluntary sector will usually be the Alzheimer's Disease Society, either through the local office or by contacting their headquarters in London.

Private sector

The private sector is beginning to provide an increasing proportion of residential and nursing care. A few private institutions also run associated day-care facilities, but not many. It is possible in some areas for families to buy in many of the other services described. This can be extremely expensive and the long-term consequences need to be considered carefully. Once started, it is very difficult to stop. Perhaps the best form of private help to buy in is the private home help to supplement that provided by the local authority, or to replace it if the latter is not available. If you can afford it, another invaluable form of help that can be hired in some areas is a private night-sitter once or twice a week. If necessary, private nursing agencies will often be able to send a nurse, but this is usually very much more expensive than coming to an arrangement with a friend or other informal carer.

Financial support

A whole range of state welfare benefits are listed in leaflets and brochures, which are available from the local social security office or very often from a post office. A social worker will also know about them, as will the local office of Age Concern, who publish their own booklet. The Alzheimer's Disease Society also has a regularly updated leaflet on welfare benefits.

There is an enormous amount of support of many different types available. It is impossible to list them all as in so many instances they have arisen in response to local demands. Some of what is available to you will be the same as elsewhere in the country, but there may well be facilities available in your area that are different to elsewhere.

Other agencies

Don't forget that a person with dementia is just as likely to need the support and input from the same range of other agencies that an undemented person may also require. These include physiotherapy if mobility becomes a problem, chiropody, a hearing assessment/aid if required, professional dental support, regular eye checks, and advice from a continence advisor if incontinence develops. Your local general practice, either through the general practitioner or a health visitor, should be able to make the appropriate arrangements.

In summary

The increasing impact of the dementias, especially Alzheimer's disease, on the lives of both the sufferers and their families has increasingly been recognized and there is now a wide range of services available from a number of different sources, for example the health service, social services, the voluntary organizations, and the private sector. The provision of such services varies enormously from one part of the country to another and trying to find out what is available locally can be a minefield. The Alzheimer's Disease Society, the Citizens' Advice Bureau, or local health visitor, and the social services department of your local authority are all there to provide information and advice, and to point you in the right direction. Don't hesitate to make use of them. The person you are concerned about is as entitled to have access to these resources as anyone else, and the same is true for you.

9

Behavioural and Psychological Problems

The behavioural and psychological problems of those suffering from dementia are often the most difficult test for those looking after them. As well as wearing a person down, constant abnormal behaviour taking the form of accusations, violence or even minor aggression, can be very hurtful and demoralizing. If a carer's sleep is continuously disturbed, it won't be long before a social crisis is precipitated. But before embarking upon individual behavioural problems, there are some general points that are worth bearing in mind and which may be relevant to many of the situations in which carers may find themselves.

We all need a routine of some sort. Some people have very regimented existences whilst others have greater flexibility in their day-to-day lives. It is very important to try to introduce a regular routine for people with dementia. This should include having a set place for objects and a set time for different activities. The dementia makes it very difficult for a person to learn new information and it can be very bewildering and frustrating to look for something that is missing, without the ability to think about where it might have been moved to. Similarly, knowing that certain activities such as mealtimes or visits to the shops generally occur at a certain time not only makes them easier to remember as the memory wanes, but can also act as a focal point which a mildly demented person can look forward to. The routine must, however, be flexible and will probably need to change as the disease advances. Once it becomes apparent that various aspects of it are not working they should not be forced upon the sufferer, but should be altered or abandoned as seems most appropriate.

In general it is best to help people with Alzheimer's disease or one of the other dementias to live as much in the real world as possible. This means regularly telling them about the environment in which they live, reminding them of the day or the month and, at least at the beginning, of the events that are going on in the world around them. However, as the disease advances, sufferers will be able to cope with this less and less and if they wish to do something unusual, there is no reason why they shouldn't as long as it isn't harmful and if it proves impossible to persuade them to do otherwise without a lot of trouble and upset. For instance, somebody I know with Alzheimer's disease insists on wearing his bathing-trunks rather than underpants. There is no harm in this and it causes much distress to both him and his wife if she tries to insist that he wears underpants.

Many people with dementia over-react to a threatening situation. This catastrophic reaction should be avoided whenever possible as it eventually does more harm than good. It may be possible to win the battle over something on one occasion but life will probably be made very much more difficult afterwards. If possible, anticipate such reactions and try to find ways around them.

While it is important to maintain the independence of individuals for as long as possible, don't try to make them undertake an activity such as doing up small buttons that you know they will not be able to complete. It is important to avoid failure as much as possible. If the activity can be managed, even though it may take two or three times as long as it would if you were to help, whenever possible it is better not to intervene but to be patient. As time goes on, however, and help is needed, rather than take over completely, start by providing assistance. Usually over a period of years the dementia will take its toll on the ability to carry out simple everyday activities and there will be a shift from independence or partial independence to more or less complete dependence. This should take place gradually and in many ways is a reverse of the situation that parents find themselves in with children. Although the situation progresses in the opposite direction, the principles are very similar.

Communication is extremely important. It is easy to attribute failure to understand what is said to the confusion that results from the dementia and think no further. Take care to speak slowly and calmly, making eye contact with the person you are addressing, and listen carefully to what they are saying. Try to give off positive rather than negative vibes, unless there is a good reason to do otherwise. If they have difficulty finding words, try to help them, but do check with them that what you have guessed is in fact correct. If a difficult situation arises make it clear that you respect the situation that they are in. If appropriate use humour to reduce tension, and if they are sad try to help them express their sadness in an understanding manner, also showing affection where this is appropriate, e.g. with a hug or by taking their hand.

In many instances, however, just as is the case in other old people, a person with dementia may have difficulty in seeing or hearing. It can be very awkward to assess the sight and hearing of a person who has an illness that causes dementia as they may be disinclined to cooperate with the assessment. Nevertheless there are all sorts of clues that can be picked up by the carer. If there is any doubt, especially with hearing, it is important to ask the doctor to examine the ears and clear out any wax. If there is still doubt, a trial with a hearing aid is often helpful in deciding whether deafness is a problem.

Communication is not confined to language, and non-verbal communication is particularly important because, as has been mentioned in earlier chapters, many of the illnesses that cause dementia interfere with a person's ability to understand and use language. Without realizing it, we all receive and transmit signals by the expressions on our faces, our gestures, and the position of our body, and the ability to respond to this type of communication is retained in many people with dementia even into the more severe stages in some cases. Smile, be positive and friendly, and don't shout unless it is necessary. You will probably have noticed how a smile usually elicits a smile in return. This often reduces tension and can help with relaxation, particularly if a difficult situation is arising. Similarly you can use the body language of the sufferer to help you understand what is going on in his or her mind. Facial expressions, actions of the hands and posture are very important. Although there are some aspects of body language that are similar in most people, individual patterns vary greatly and if you observe carefully you can soon learn to pick up the signs.

As well as speaking clearly, and in some cases slowly, and using relatively simple language, it is often a good idea to use props when trying to communicate with someone who is beginning to have difficulty with language. Photographs of members of the family or friends and pointing to the individual when discussing them can be helpful, as can the use of large calendars or clocks for the purpose of time-orientation. Disorientation in space is often another problem and some families that I know have painted the doors in their house in different colours to help distinguish between the kitchen and the dining room. You can take this a step further by putting a picture on the door, of a WC or a bed as appropriate.

For the highest standards of care, the important points are to establish a routine, but to treat this flexibly as the situation will change; to make the most of communication, both verbal and non-verbal; to avoid catastrophic over-reactions; to avoid situations that cause a sense of failure; and to be protective without being over-protective. In other words you will need to be a paragon of all the virtues, which is of course impossible. It is important to accept this and to realize that you may sometimes appear to make mistakes, but as long as you are trying to do the best you can, that is all anyone can really expect of you.

Social situations

One of the earliest problems that relatives have to cope with is embarrassing behaviour in the presence of friends or others. This is most likely to occur if the event is taking place away from a familiar environment such as the home. Large parties ought probably to be avoided. Having to relate to a continual stream of different people can be very threatening and bewildering. This may well provoke anger and frustration. It is important nevertheless to try to maintain some social interaction and this is best managed by inviting a few friends or relatives to your own home, having first explained the situation. You can also advise them in advance about appropriate topics of conversation – things to do with the past, for example, if the dementia has progressed to the stage where there is no longer any interest in or memory for current events. It is particularly important to ask the visitor not to exclude the person with dementia from the conversation.

For as long as table manners are preserved there is no reason why a small and friendly group should not eat out in a quiet restaurant or pub. Visits to the theatre and cinema may also be possible for a while, but in the later stages of illness the dimly lit environment may cause problems as may a desire to relate to whatever is happening on the screen or stage.

Holidays

When it becomes apparent that a person's memory is failing and that he or she is becoming muddled, relatives often feel that a good holiday will sort the situation out. This is not always a good idea. Not only will routine be disturbed, but the environment will be completely unfamiliar and all sorts of problems can arise. These range from incontinence because of an inability to find the bathroom in the middle of the night, even if it adjoins the bedroom, to emotional outbursts of either anger or tears. Many relatives have had to abandon a holiday after only a few days and return home.

Although I know of several elderly people who have successfully taken their husband or wife with Alzheimer's disease abroad, air travel should only be attempted with much caution and probably only in the earlier stages of dementia. The cramped confines of an aircraft, the strange activities that appear to go on, and loss of touch with reality frequently cause problems. One elderly man with multiple infarct dementia, while watching the in-flight movie, decided that he had had enough, didn't like what he was watching, and wanted to go home. His wife thought that he was going to the toilet, which was just the other side of the gangway. Unfortunately he suddenly realized that he couldn't see the exit, panicked, and caused a lot of distress to himself, his wife and other passengers.

A safe and secure environment with which they feel familiar is much more important for people with dementia than a holiday.

Wandering

At some stage in their illness many people with dementia will show a tendency to wander. This can be a problem even if it is confined to the house, but some people will take to wandering, sometimes miles, away from home. Because this is potentially dangerous it usually causes a lot of anxiety and distress for the carers. It is, however, almost impossible to be absolutely certain that you could prevent a wanderer from 'escaping'. Even in a hospital it isn't feasible to watch someone for twenty-four hours a day.

There seem to be many different types of wandering and it is a form of abnormal behaviour that is only just beginning to be studied in detail. In some people with dementia it may result from boredom, in others perhaps it is a way of using up an excess of energy; on occasions it may be a reaction to pain or discomfort. In many cases it seems that sufferers are looking for somebody or something, for instance trying to find the house they lived in when they were a child under the mistaken impression that it is still their home. At a simpler level, some people wander when they have been moved into a new environment and once they become familiar with the layout of the accommodation and settle into a routine, the wandering will cease.

Another quite common cause of wandering is the mistaken impression sufferers can have that they have an appointment or that the time for an appointment has arrived when it may not in fact be for several hours, or may even be on an entirely different day.

There are various ways of trying to tackle wandering. If it is at all possible it is worth making an effort to understand the reason behind it. This means that one has to be certain that there is no additional medical problem that is causing distress and medical advice may have to be sought. If, however, boredom seems to be at the root of the matter, then increased activity may well help. Very often all that one can do is to divert the person's attention to some other activity that doesn't involve wandering. When disturbed in the middle of the night, some carers suggest that the sufferer has a cup of tea before he or she leaves for wherever they imagine they are going. Whilst the tea is made, it is often possible to divert attention away from leaving the house to something else and from there to the need to go to bed. If they insist on leaving the house, particularly if they appear to be becoming aggressive or violent, it is best to let them leave, to accompany them, and to try to divert their attention while walking so that they will eventually come round the block with you back to home.

Unfortunately a determined wanderer will sometimes escape. There is no reason why you can't fit suitable locks and bolts to the doors, but do make sure that they are not difficult to open in the case of an emergency, for example a fire. Give your relative an identity bracelet or some other means of identification, including your telephone number or that of a neighbour if you don't have a telephone of your own. Make sure that local people, neighbours and shopkeepers for example, know of the problem so that they can alert you if necessary.

If, despite all precautions, the sufferer wanders off for some time, undetected and unseen by anybody, don't panic. Accidents happen very rarely. I can think of hundreds of people with dementia who have wandered regularly, despite the best efforts of those caring for them, yet I only know of two or three who suffered in consequence. The greatest difficulty caused by wandering is the reluctance of day centres and nursing homes to take responsibility for a person who may disappear. This naturally increases the stress on those caring for them. Drugs are usually of little help, but may have to be tried as a last resort. It is essential though that they are only used for a short period and withdrawn very early if they don't appear to be helping.

Problems at night

Those suffering from a dementia may well disturb other people's sleep. Sometimes it is because they have a tendency to wander; sometimes they are disorientated and think that it is time to get up; sometimes they are frightened at night. Often, having gone to the bathroom they are unable to find their way back to the bedroom or have their attention diverted to something else with which they then become involved.

Many people with dementia are less active than they used to be during the daytime and may even take more daytime naps than before. Try to make sure they get adequate physical and mental activity during the day, to help promote sleep. It is also a good idea to try to ensure that they go to the bathroom last thing before going to bed; restricting fluids during the evening, say after supper if this does not cause distress, can also help. Leaving a light on in the bathroom and having a low-wattage bulb on the landing can assist a confused person in getting around at night.

The bed needs to be comfortable and some relatives find that continental quilts are easier for a person with dementia to manage than blankets and sheets. It is probably best not to use cot sides as they rarely manage to deter a wanderer and can be irritating. Sometimes, however, they can be helpful in preventing a person from falling out of bed if this is a problem.

If sufferers decide to get dressed and you have difficulty dissuading them, don't worry – let them get on with it. They may well be prepared to go back to bed, even though fully clothed. Sometimes a warm drink works as it is often associated with the going-to-bed routine.

Finally, there are two important points. First, if wandering at night is a real problem, make sure there are no hazards to safety, like gas taps that could be turned on. Second, a step that can be taken is to ask the doctor to prescribe some sleeping medicines. These should be avoided except as a last resort and should only be tried for a few weeks at a time. Sometimes it can be left to the carer's discretion to administer them intermittently, perhaps after having had two or three bad nights in a row. All medicines have side-effects and you must ask the doctor what to watch out for if they were to affect the person you are looking after.

Restlessness and agitation

Many people with dementia, especially Alzheimer's disease, become restless, anxious and agitated. They may pace nervously up and down, talk incessantly, or fidget. This can be very wearing to carers. Sometimes it is a side-effect of medicines, but not very often. The medicines most commonly responsible are sedatives that belong to the group known as *phenothiazines*. The doctor who prescribes them should be aware of this side-effect, and warn you to be on the look-out for it.

Often the restlessness and agitation are a response to an inappropriate belief. An elderly patient of mine thought she was living in her boarding-school and couldn't understand why her mother hadn't come to fetch her to take her home for the summer holiday. She was under the impression that she was alone in the school, having been there for several days after all her friends and the teachers had left. She was understandably very upset and very agitated. This happened frequently, usually at about eleven o'clock in the morning.

If a situation like this arises, try to be reassuring. You may have to enter into the spirit of the misbelief and, for instance, take some of the responsibility away from the mind of the sufferer by saying that you will look after whatever it is that is causing the concern.

When the distressing behaviour occurs at a regular time, it may be possible to break the cycle, for instance by making sure that the sufferer is otherwise engaged in an activity at the appropriate time. If this doesn't work, try a walk or a drive together or a visit to a neighbour. After attempting this diversional therapy for a few days or sometimes a little longer, you may find that the problem doesn't recur. If it does, try to establish a different routine that regularly diverts attention away from other matters to something specific at this particular time.

If fidgeting is a problem – the constant rearrangement of decorations on the mantelpiece and so on – provide something else to fidget with. Worry beads, a few coins or a piece of string are amongst the things that some relatives have successfully managed to substitute for a more generalized fidgety behaviour. If absolutely essential, drugs can again be tried as a last resort.

Losing track of time

Eventually many if not all people with dementia will lose track of time. This can lead to many difficulties for relatives and carers. A sufferer may well forget when he or she last ate, when bedtime is, accuse you of having been away for hours when in fact you have only been absent for a few minutes, and so on. It can be very difficult to cope with, especially if you need to go out and leave him or her alone.

Sometimes drawing a clock-face with the time for lunch or some other activity represented by the position of the hands is helpful. This will only work, however, if the sufferer has the ability to compare the diagram with the time displayed on a clock. It is probably better to have a simple clock with a large face. In many ways a digital clock may seem easier, but in my experience the old-fashioned type is superior for people with dementia.

An old-fashioned egg-timer-type hour-glass may be a useful device. It needs to be fairly robust, but you can tell the sufferer that you will be back, that lunch will happen, or that the programme on television will start when the sand has all gone from the top to the bottom.

Sexual behaviour

This can be a problem for two reasons. Sometimes a person with dementia becomes sexually more active than is socially acceptable. On the other hand many partners still have sexual needs of their own. If the carer still feels the need for sexual relations with the husband or wife, there is of course absolutely nothing wrong with this and it may be possible to obtain the appropriate responses even though the carer may need to take the initiative.

Sometimes a person with dementia, especially if it is caused by a condition like Pick's disease, may lose the normal sexual inhibitions that we all learn earlier in life and make inappropriate advances to others. This can of course be very embarrassing and distressing to the object of attention and also to the carers. This type of behaviour should be very definitely but very gently discouraged, as should masturbation in public.

If a person with dementia appears naked unexpectedly or undresses in public, there is probably no sexual connotation to this at all. A man may start to fiddle with his trousers and take them off because he feels the need to relieve himself, but has forgotten that he should first go to the bathroom and that he should not undress in front of other people. It is very important not to over-react to situations like this, but to explain gently to him what he should and shouldn't do and to undertake this in a manner which will be interpreted as providing assistance rather than anger.

One elderly lady with Alzheimer's disease kept lifting her skirt up when other people were present and, if unchecked, began to pull down her underwear. This appeared to be because she was under the impression, often mistakenly, that she needed to pass urine. Her husband successfully overcame this by dressing her in trousers when they were in the company of others and these trousers had a Velcro fastener at the back. Being unable to adapt easily to new things, she soon stopped trying to remove the trousers as she couldn't work out how to undo the fastening. Instead she intimated to her husband from time to time that something was amiss, prompting him to take her to the bathroom when necessary.

The loss of a physical relationship, or a change in this that makes it unsatisfactory, can cause emotional problems to those who are caring for a spouse with a dementia. Sometimes these can be very difficult to come to terms with, or find the best way of adapting to. Despite the fact that many people find it very difficult to talk about their sexual feelings, it is important that this aspect of a relationship is taken seriously, and your doctor, or other health professional if you are in contact with one, e.g. a community psychiatric nurse, may be able to suggest a trained counsellor. Although this will not change the situation, it may nevertheless be helpful. Before embarking upon a course of counselling, however, do ask how much you will have to pay.

Suspiciousness

Some people with dementia are very unpleasant to those around them. They may accuse a spouse of trying to harm them, of stealing their belongings, of plotting against them, and so on. This type of behaviour is really very upsetting and often causes deep hurt. There is little one can do about it, as no amount of reasoning will make any long-term difference. In the short-term, however, reassurance can sometimes be helpful, as the outburst may really be a means of saying 'I don't feel loved' or 'I am angry because I am frightened'. If this type of emotional insecurity is responsible, loving reassurance and a hug may well be the answer, but don't feel rejected if this doesn't work. There must be many other reasons for a reaction of this nature and the underlying cause is often not apparent. Very often all that one can do is to try to ignore such comments and remember that they are not really the expression of a considered thought, but the results of brain damage. The sufferer is probably as upset and distressed about the situation as the person to whom the remarks are directed.

Above all, don't try to react by justifying yourself or arguing. This could well result in a catastrophic reaction. If the situation has arisen because the sufferer has forgotten who a person is, even though they should know them quite well, and mistakes them for a stranger who, for instance, could be a thief, try to explain the situation to the other person or persons involved and at the same time reassure the sufferer.

If things get lost, it is very likely that they have either been put down in a strange place or that they have been deliberately hidden. You will soon learn about the favourite hiding-places. This will help you to recover things quickly when the sufferer begins to complain that they have disappeared and has forgotten that he or she has hidden them. If a lockable drawer or cupboard is the hiding-place have duplicate keys made or remove the existing key in case objects are locked away and the key in turn is hidden elsewhere or lost. It is also a good idea to keep objects such as jewellery, cash, legal documents, and so on safely away from a demented person in case they too disappear.

Repetition

Just as loss of the sense of time with consequent repeated questioning can be very wearing, so can repeated questioning about other matters. It is often something that you can't do anything about, as no matter how much reassurance you provide and no matter how many times you answer the questions, they will continue to be asked. It may result from just the memory loss but there is often a background of insecurity and the need for constant reassurance.

Sometimes writing down the answer to a complex question on a piece of paper or on a blackboard can be helpful, as the sufferer can then be diverted to the answer without the need for a lengthy explanation, particularly if the situation is a complex one. More usually, however, the question is a simple one with a simple answer and writing things down just creates additional work and does little to help relieve the situation. Under these circumstances it is best to arrange to escape from time to time, to give yourself breathing-space. If you detect that the repetitive questioning is really a need for reassurance based upon a feeling of insecurity, perhaps provide feedback in the form of love and affection at times when it is not being sought and no questions are being asked. If the questioner's needs are only fulfilled in response to repeated questioning, this reinforces the pattern. If, however, the sufferer appreciates that he or she is loved and wanted and that this is true without having to seek attention, the questioning may occur less frequently.

Hallucinations

Hallucinations – seeing or hearing people, voices, or things that aren't really there – often happen as a result of dementia. It can be very frightening, both for the sufferer and the carer. Some people with dementia form quite a close attachment to their 'invisible friend' but more often than not the experience is a distressing one. This situation is best handled by reassurance. Explain that you know they can see someone who you can't and try to be supportive. Whatever happens, don't try to tell them that they are wrong, and that there is no one there. To them the hallucination is very real, and it is important that they know that you appreciate the situation that they are in.

Sometimes visual hallucinations result from either a false impression given by an inadequately lit and dimly perceived object or from poor sight. If the illumination in the room appears poor, improve it and see whether this helps.

If hallucinations become a major problem it is important to seek medical advice, as this is one situation where medication may actually be helpful. There is, however, no point in treating them unless they are causing distress or upset or are disrupting the daily routine.

A similar problem, although not really a hallucination, can occur when people with dementia see their own reflection in a mirror. They may fail to realize that it is their own image they are seeing and interpret their reflection as indicating the presence of a stranger. This can sometimes provoke an aggressive or fearful response. If this is a particular problem, a small curtain or cloth can be draped across the mirror, enabling others to use it when necessary, whilst at the same time removing the cause of the distress.

Depression

Many people with dementia become depressed. This can be the result of a realization, usually early on in the course of the disease, that their brain isn't working as it should. Sometimes it happens for other reasons and occasionally an apparent dementia can, in fact, be depression. There is a difference between being depressed and feeling miserable. A person who is depressed will usually be withdrawn and unhappy, will speak, act and think slowly. This can affect the daily routine and interest in food, and is sometimes associated with early morning awakening with difficulty in getting back to sleep. Some people with depression experience mood swings, and are much happier in the evening than they are when they first get up in the morning.

If depression is present against a background of dementia, it can be difficult to realize that the increased impairment in the sufferer's intellectual ability is the result of depression rather than of a worsening of the dementing process. If you ever have any fears that the sufferer has depression, it is best to ask the doctor for advice. He should be able to help, even if he has to refer the sufferer to a psychiatrist for a more expert assessment.

The presence of depression will often mean that the sufferer requires even more love and support. If he or she is given medicine for the depression, this may actually cause a worsening of the memory for a while and may have other side-effects, depending upon the type of medicine prescribed. It is important that you ask the doctor to let you know what you should be looking out for, and also important to decide whether the treatment seems worthwhile. In some patients, anti-depressants, especially the older types, can just make the situation worse. Nevertheless, it is often necessary to undertake a few weeks' trial of the treatment, just to see whether there is any improvement.

One very important thing not to forget is that one mustn't expect someone with depression to 'snap out of it'. A person with normal intellectual function can't manage this and it is even less possible for someone with dementia. Depression is an illness that has a physical basis to it and is not just an attitude of mind. It has to be regarded in the same light as other medical illnesses that are more clearly due to physical abnormality.

Aggression

Some people with dementia can become extremely aggressive, but most do not. Although spouses are often very expert at managing the aggression if it occurs, the involvement of children can be a very serious problem. An aggressive or violent, confused adult can cause major distress to children and even teenagers who don't understand what is going on. When children are affected it is a natural reaction to become angry with the sufferer, but although the situation must be resolved, it is important not to lose sight of the fact that the aggression is not a conscious, considered action of the sufferer. It results from brain damage and something has triggered off an abnormal behavioural response. This 'something' may be a misinterpretation of events going on around the sufferer, a feeling of inadequacy that is exaggerated by the attitude of younger people, or a hundred and one other things. The main thing is to stay calm and this will usually be a help to other people. As is the case with so many other abnormalities of behaviour in these circumstances, the best approach is often that of diversion, distracting attention in another direction and gently persuading the sufferer to become interested in an alternative activity.

Try and work out what it is that might be precipitating the outbursts and hope to avoid similar situations in the future. Above all, if this type of behaviour becomes a real problem, seek advice earlier rather than later. Very rarely, aggressive behaviour is consistently directed against one person for no obvious reason, with threats of harm or even expressions of intent to kill. This situation has arisen many times, but actual physical violence occurs exceptionally rarely. Nevertheless, it is absolutely essential that a carer seeks support and help as soon as they find themselves threatened. Having to live in fear of being attacked will affect not only carers, but also their relationship with the demented relative. Aggressive behaviour can usually be treated successfully by the careful administration of medicines.

Never react to violence with violence or anger, as this won't prevent a further occurrence; try to avoid aggressive situations developing and step back out of reach if there is any obvious evidence that you are about to be assaulted. If threats of physical harm become a reality, seek medical help at the first opportunity. Remember, it is always better to try to prevent aggressive situations from developing, so try to learn the warning signs and try to avoid situations that you know may precipitate aggression. Finally, remember that the aggression is not under the control of the person with dementia, and it would not be helpful to try and 'get your own back' or punish them for their actions, as this will often make the situation worse.

Safety

People who cannot think properly for themselves are far more likely to have accidents that the rest of us would be able to avoid. It is important to lock away poisons and medicines, to be wary of gas stoves and fires, and to take care over hot objects or those containing boiling water or other fluids. Trailing flexes, loose mats and other hazards of this type should be tidied up and it may be necessary to put locks on certain doors and windows. Take particular care if a person with dementia is a smoker – never leave him or her alone with cigarettes or pipe tobacco and matches. Make sure that the hot water in your system isn't so hot that it can burn skin, if hands are unwarily plunged into a basinful, or a person steps into a bathful. Ensure that your home has adequate lighting and leave a landing light on at night if the person with dementia is in the habit of getting up, whether to go to the toilet or for any other reason.

If the stairs are a potential hazard, especially at night, consider installing a gate at the top, possibly with an attached alarm that will let you know when it is being opened. A similar gate may also be helpful at the bottom of the stairs. Make sure that the hand rails on the stairs are adequate and if there aren't any, you should think of installing some, as they can often be grabbed at the last moment if a person becomes unsteady.

Most accidents happen in the kitchen, with the stairs and the bathroom following closely behind. Think carefully about your own and ask relatives of other people with dementia about their experiences. It is better to take precautions to prevent an accident rather than have to cope with the consequences of one. Both the gas and the electricity boards are aware of the problems posed by people with dementia and will advise and help in making cookers, fires, and other equipment safe. Rails around the toilet and near the handbasin, and non-slip mats in the bath or shower, are also a good investment.

Lastly, don't forget that you too will be more prone to accidents. It is well established that people who are living under additional stress and strain, constantly rushing to get things done and often exhausted from lack of sleep, are much more likely to have an accident. It is very important to take care of yourself.

10

Looking After Yourself

Many people who are caring for a relative with dementia are tempted to struggle on, as independently as possible, for as long as they possibly can, with as little help as possible and with as little change in their normal pattern of life as possible. Despite the understandable motivation behind such an approach, it often ends in disaster. Instead of one person to look after, the health service or the social services may then have two. In addition, the toll exacted of carers may be so great that it prevents them from carrying on, irrespective of how much help and support they can be offered. The personal and emotional costs of caring for a person with dementia are enormous and all carers need to realize this as it will help them plan for the future. One of the biggest problems is coming to terms with one's own emotional reactions and responses to one of the most demanding tasks that can be thrust upon us.

Guilt

For many people, guilt is the most destructive of all the emotions aroused by caring for a person with dementia. It can undermine the carer's self-esteem and can arise, initially, as a consequence of choosing a course of action deemed best for the sufferer. On the one hand the family may decide to have an elderly parent living with them, so that they can care for him or her; on the other they may decide that the sufferer would be best looked after in a hospital or a home. In each situation the carers will believe that the path they have chosen is best for their relative, either because they are preventing them having to live in an institution or because they are avoiding the need for them to live at home where everybody else in the house may be out at work or school, for example.

So often, both approaches result in considerable guilt. The family that have decided to entrust the care of their relative with dementia to an institution feel guilty about not looking after him or her themselves, while the family who have elected to keep their relative at home may worry that by providing such a high standard of care they have prolonged a life that is causing distress to the sufferer and may also have introduced all sorts of stresses and strains into the family that they never dreamed would occur. Whatever you do is likely to appear to be wrong at some time. There are very few situations to which there is only one correct answer – in most you have to accept the best compromise, and this will vary very much from family to family. It has to be remembered that by the very nature of compromise, there are bound to be disadvantages to the chosen course of action.

Many of the other problems that are mentioned in this chapter – anger, changing family responsibilities, the possibility of your own physical illness, sexual relationships, and so on – may well make you feel guilty and undermine your self-confidence. As with so many other similar positions it is impossible to come to terms with such a problem and live with it until you realize what is happening and can accept it. In these circumstances you also have to accept that you are in a no-win situation and as long as you know that you are doing the best that you can, that is all that anyone can expect of you. It is essential that you break free from your own particular circle of guilt as much as you possibly can and don't allow it to stop you thinking positively about the future.

Guilt that is festering inside can be very damaging. You may not wish to talk to other people about it, either because you are too ashamed to admit that you feel guilty because of something that has happened or because you feel they won't understand your own emotional responses. This is where counselling can be very helpful, whether in the form of attending a support group or on a more individual basis, and discussing the problem with others who have either faced the same problem themselves or worked very closely with families in a similar situation in the past.

You may at times be embarrassed by the behaviour of your relative with dementia, whether this involves something dramatic like screaming in public or forgetting to pay for things in a shop, or more minor problems like poor table manners which are apparent to other people. Incontinence and changing sexuality also cause embarrassment. Many carers feel guilty about their own embarrassment, but this is a situation that you should be able to tackle. Explaining the situation to others involved and asking them to make allowances would be much more helpful than trying to pretend that nothing is happening or that you don't know what is going on. Sharing the problem, where this is possible, will often relieve the tension and sense of embarrassment. This in itself will help alleviate the degree of guilt that may be felt. So it should be possible in some but not all situations that are potentially embarrassing to reduce the feeling of guilt by reducing the extent of the embarrassment.

Arranging for a relative with dementia to be admitted to a home or a hospital, even for a short period, is one of the situations that often arouses the greatest feelings of guilt. Even if a break is desperately needed or you have been caring for your relative for years and really have got to the end of the road, the feeling of relief is so often mingled with one of shame at having apparently abandoned him or her to the care of others. If the admission is a short-term one, to allow you to recharge your batteries, being advised to stay away, or go away on holiday so that you have a complete break, may also make this worse. It is important, however, to put each of these situations in the correct context.

As far as a short-term admission is concerned, this is the sufferer's side of the contract. In return for being able to continue living at home the sufferer has to accept, albeit unknowingly, some of the consequences of the unsatisfactory nature of the compromise that has been forced upon all involved. A short-term admission to allow the carer some relief is after all in the sufferer's best interest. It will usually result in him or her being able to stay at home for longer and even if he or she is distressed while away from home, and disturbed for a while afterwards, the memory will soon fade.

When institutional care has had to be arranged on a permanent basis, whether in a hospital or in a private home, there is no need to feel a sense of abandoning the sufferer. The need usually arises after the carers have done all they can to cope for as long as possible and when, because of their own particular circumstances, and possibly others relating to the sufferer, they can no longer provide the necessary level of care. At this point, the sufferer is usually best looked after by people with professional skills. The fact that some families manage to continue caring at home until the end of the illness should not make others feel guilty if they are unable to do the same. Circumstances are never the same and we are all made differently; some people can cope more effectively with particular situations than others and some dementia sufferers are much more difficult to cope with than others.

There is also no need to feel that you are abandoning the sufferer if you continue to visit him or her on a regular basis while it still seems to you that you are eliciting some kind of response. For many dementia sufferers, however, the time will come when it is no longer important who looks after them, but essential that they are looked after in the best way possible. Social interaction is eventually reduced for many, although not all, dementia sufferers and there will come a time when regular visiting may seem less important. If this situation does arise, it is still important to visit from time to time for the sake of the professional carers who have taken over. It will also enable you to keep in touch with what is going on and to be happy that as much as can be done is being done.

Anger

You will often feel angry and may at times perhaps even feel violent. Many a carer has almost physically attacked, and some even actually attacked, the person they are looking after. This is a natural reaction and we all have our own tolerance level. Your anger will be very mixed – it will be directed at the sufferer, directed at yourself for having reacted in the way that you have, and directed at the general situation that has allowed these circumstances to prevail. You may be angry with the doctors for not being able to cure the dementia, with others for not providing adequate services, with the government for not making better care available, and so on.

When this situation arises – and if it hasn't it almost certainly will – try to remember that the behaviour that has provoked it is not aimed at you as an individual, but is a response engendered within the sufferer by his or her illness. However personal an attack on you it may appear to be, it is merely a symptom of the sufferer's illness.

If you arrive at the point of only just being able to stop yourself being physically aggressive or have actually been unable to prevent yourself responding in this way, you need help and support. It is not something to be ashamed of, it is not something to lock up inside yourself; it is a warning to everybody that you need help. To whom you turn will depend very much on your own circumstances. Other members of the family may be able to help relieve the strain, either by taking over for a while or by acting as an emotional outlet. A friend in a similar position to yourself, perhaps met through a support group, may also be able to help. You ought, anyway, to visit your doctor as he may be able to mobilize professional support that will sustain you in the longer term. Please try not to feel ashamed and guilty; your reaction is normal and everybody has their breaking point. Once you have discovered yours, you should try to plan ahead. In some ways your task may be easier for knowing where you stand. Also, remember that whatever you have done, the sufferer will almost certainly forget, unless it is a repeated and frequent occurrence.

Paradoxically, like so many other situations in life, it is the apparently trivial situations that cause the greatest problems. For this reason you may not feel like sharing your problem with others, but it is important that you overcome this reluctance. If you can also manage to distinguish between your anger at the sufferer's behaviour and your anger with the person himself or herself, this may make your burden easier to bear.

A sense of 'living bereavement'

As a dementing illness progresses, relatives and, to a lesser extent, friends have to come to terms with the loss of someone they love. Although this process is a slow one, starting with the realization that the sufferer is not the person he or she used to be, and progressing to a loss of companionship and a hundred and one other losses, it is very much akin to the grief and bereavement experienced after someone has died. Although the body is physically still present, the personality goes. This is particularly painful when the sufferer is unable to communicate with, understand, or recognize you. This sense of loss is very difficult to cope with sometimes, and the long-drawn-out grieving process may affect the pattern of bereavement when the sufferer eventually dies. Just as you come to terms with the situation, your relative may deteriorate in another way and you have to adjust all over again.

With a progressive illness like dementia, the grief can get worse as time goes on and very often death is a merciful release from this type of emotional turmoil, just as it is from the physical burdens and the distressful existence of the sufferer. Many people won't understand what you are going through. We can all relate to the recently bereaved, but this is a situation that is only really understood by others who have experienced it, either first-hand or by working closely with those in your position. As for so many of the emotional problems that arise when caring for a person with dementia, the main anchor in coping with the living bereavement process can only be a sharing of the experience with others. There is little to be gained from keeping a stiff upper lip and maintaining a façade of emotional independence.

Family problems

Coping with dementia can generate two different types of family problem. The first is the stress that can be caused by the demands that the disease process makes on the carers, and often their children. The second, connected with the first, is the ill-feeling that can sometimes be fostered within families because one or two members feel that they are taking most, if not all, of the responsibility and providing the greater part of the care.

It is important that all members of the family are involved in making decisions about the pattern of care that is to be provided and the support that is required. If you are a lone carer among others who are helping only a little or not at all, it may help to arrange a family conference so that they all are aware of how you are feeling and what you are having to cope with. If you are beginning to feel that you have gone as far as you can on your own, make this plain in a sensitive way and ask the others not just whether they can help, but how they can help. If the time has come when lack of additional support means the sufferer will have to go into an institution, for example, they have to realize that this is a family decision and not just yours. You have done all that you can and they are saying that they have done all that they can. Even if you are the mainstay of the care that is being given to your relative with dementia, it is not just you that is responsible for any change in the pattern of care, but all your family together. In other words, the change is occurring not just because you can't carry on but because they can't help either. Above all, don't carry on nurturing ill feelings beneath an apparently unworried outward appearance. Dementia is a family disease, and the whole family has a responsibility to anyone suffering from it.

When younger relatives take an aged parent with dementia into their household, this often has an impact on their own children. Children can suffer anything from the loss of their bedroom to less personal attention from their parents, though they tend to be remarkably good at coping with situations like this and adapt very well. It is often the parents' worries on behalf of their children that are the problem, rather than the effect on the children themselves. Sometimes, however, children can be affected adversely and there is no way of predicting this in advance. Fear, particularly in younger children, can often be overcome by explaining what is going on and why their grandparent is now so different, and also letting them see how you handle situations and relate to their grandparent. Very often children form a delightful relationship with a demented elderly person, particularly in the earlier stages of dementia, and this is probably beneficial to all involved. Children's love can be very different from that of adults – a natural expression of affection rather than a feeling of duty, which is so often a part of the emotional relationship between an adult and his or her ageing parent.

The biggest problems usually involve teenagers. They may be embarrassed to bring their friends into their home and feel isolated as a result; they can feel reluctant to let their friends know the situation, in case they become the object of ridicule. There may also be clashes, either because they are asked to help or because although they would like to, it would conflict with the demands made upon them by the usual teenage activities. It is very important that they understand what is going on; sometimes, as in the case with younger children, teenagers can make a major and very positive contribution to the care of a person with dementia. There is an excellent book by Jane Gilliard – *The Long and Winding Road: A Young Person's Guide to Dementia* – which is specifically aimed at helping young people overcome the problems that they will encounter when a member of their family is diagnosed with dementia. This should be available from your local bookshop; it is published by Wrightson Biomedical Publishing Limited.

It is essential, when accepting an older person with dementia into your home, not to expect that the whole family should arrange their lives around the sufferer. The other family members will still need time and attention from each other, possibly even more so than before, and everyone will have to be very sensitive about one another's needs. Hostility or aggression in one member of the family should not be allowed to spread; rather, the underlying stresses and strains should, if possible, be addressed.

In some cases, despite the best of intentions, taking a relative with dementia into the family home is disastrous. If this happens, you have to rest content with the knowledge that you have at least tried to do the best that you can. It is important not to feel guilty about exploring alternative approaches to care. It is the integrity of your own immediate family that is most important. If this breaks up, not only will the sufferer lose out, but so will everybody else. Take seriously any tendency to arguments and family unhappiness before it goes too far.

Changing responsibilities

The onset of dementia in a person changes all sorts of roles within the family, from the more obvious 'children caring for parents' situation to that in which a spouse has to take on the role traditionally undertaken in their family by the sufferer until he or she became ill. The role of physical carer can be a particularly difficult one to cope with; as the disease progresses, of course, the level of care needed will become greater, not less.

For most older people it has been traditional for the husband to run the family's financial affairs. Many older women have little idea of the complexity of what often seemed like simple financial details. Similarly, for a man to have to take on the role of the housewife, the cooking, cleaning, shopping, washing, and so on, can prove very difficult. All these activities are simple if you have been doing them for forty or fifty years as they have become second nature. To have to start from scratch and learn to undertake your spouse's role, as well as carry on with your own, and at the same time adjust to all the emotional and other problems of coping for a person with dementia, is a pretty tall order and I sometimes marvel at how well most people cope. To those of us on the outside, preparing a meal or checking a bank statement seems simple, and on their own they may be, but one has to remember that all this must be viewed in the overall context of the impact that dementia makes not just on the sufferer, but on the family too.

Of all the problems that arise it is often the role reversal between child and parent that creates most difficulty. Some children find it very nearly impossible to help one of their parents undertake the basic activities of life, such as washing and bathing, going to the toilet, and cleaning up afterwards. On the other hand, as far as spouses are concerned, one has to remember that it is easier to learn how to undertake practical tasks than it is to take on responsibility for making important decisions that may affect the future. It is up to individual members of a family to learn to help each other in circumstances like this. What may be a monumentally difficult task for an older person to take on may be of little consequence to a younger member of the family or to a brother or sister living near by. A son, for instance, could shop for parents as well as himself or take responsibility for financial matters. It is also possible to get help from the statutory services with some of the more practical tasks such as keeping the house clean and preparing food. Talk to other people who have managed to cope with a similar experience; they may well be able to point the way ahead.

Finally, it is important not to underestimate the effect that this role reversal has upon the sufferers. They may experience an acute sense of failure when they realize they can no longer undertake a task adequately and that someone else has taken on responsibility for it. Whenever possible, continue to involve them for as long as is practical. They may then still feel part of the system and if you can sustain this approach for long enough, the point at which they can no longer be involved may occur at a stage in the illness when they are also unlikely to realize what has happened or be able to worry about it.

Isolation

Many carers feel extremely isolated when the immensity of the task ahead dawns on them. Some have struggled on for years before realizing that many people are in a similar position to themselves. The isolation is not just psychological, but also physical. Some sufferers with dementia require almost constant attendance, twenty-four hours a day. This gives little opportunity for a carer, particularly an elderly spouse who may have physical problems of his or her own, to get out and meet other people, other than the occasional short trip to the shops. Social activities often take second place to what appear to be more essential daily tasks. The situation is often compounded by embarrassment at the behavioural abnormalities that so frequently occur. If the doctor or other professionals are found to be caring, supportive, and understanding of the carer's predicament, they may themselves help to break the feeling of isolation and at the same time point a carer in the direction of additional forms of help.

Many people find themselves in a situation where it is the very person to whom they would have turned for help that has developed the dementia. This can be a particularly cruel predicament and it is essential that a carer in this situation makes contact with others, either through a support group, a day hospital, a day centre, or via family and friends. In particular, discover what type of day-care and sitting-in services are available in your area, which will enable you to break free and meet other people.

Sexual relationships

Many people still find it difficult to discuss sexual matters even within a normal and loving relationship. When one partner has dementia it can seem totally inappropriate and perhaps wrong to even think about such things. This is a mistake. Most people, if not everybody, need loving, physical contact, both sexual and otherwise.

Often people with dementia can remain affectionate for some considerable period into the course of their illness. They may well respond to the same cues as they have done in the past, the familiarity of which may give them confidence and satisfaction. Sometimes, however, sexual responses change, the physical side of a relationship lapses, and the matter is buried in an attempt to relegate it to the subconscious.

As mentioned before, taking a more active role may help, but usually this is only beneficial in the earlier stages of the illness. The sexual and physical aspects of a relationship are such a personal and intimate part of one's life that it is unlikely a carer will wish to talk about them, other than with a specially trained counsellor. Some doctors may be able to help, but few are trained in this field. They should, however, be able to help you contact a person with the appropriate training.

For many people, sexual intercourse itself is not what is missed most. It is the physical and asexual expression of an affectionate relationship that means so much.

Falling ill yourself

Many people looking after an older person with dementia are themselves elderly and suffer with chronic medical conditions of one sort or another. If on top of these they also have to cope with the mental and physical demands of caring for someone with dementia, it is possible that their own illnesses may be aggravated. Many have to struggle on despite being unwell themselves.

If, however, a carer is really laid low with a medical problem or has an accident, such as a fractured hip, somebody else is going to have to look after the sufferer. If possible, try to avoid a social crisis at the last minute by making contingency plans, ensuring that your general practitioner is aware of them or better still has helped in drawing them up. Many carers can call upon family and friends in emergencies such as this, as long as there is no likelihood of a protracted, drawn-out illness.

If at all possible, it is always better for sufferers from dementia to remain in their own home, even if their normal routine is broken and people with whom they are less familiar are there to look after them. If this arrangement looks unlikely to work, it is probable that admission to a hospital or a home will have to be organized, at least in the short term.

What happens if the carer collapses unconscious and is unable to call for help? This situation does not arise very often, but sometimes it does and many people, particularly older spouses, worry about it. The best way of coping with this is to arrange for someone to look in regularly, once or twice a day, and to give them the means to report back to a third person, usually another member of the family or a doctor, if anything seems amiss. The unavoidable intrusion into the carer's life-style has to be balanced against the advantages of such a scheme. An alternative approach is to use the telephone to make regular daily contact.

There is also the possibility that a carer may fall without losing consciousness, but be unable to summon help. A person with dementia may well be incapable of helping in these circumstances and can sometimes make matters worse. Having a pendant or wrist-watch alarm system will usually instil a feeling of confidence and will be of practical benefit should the need arise. These systems usually consist of a small box, about the size of a wrist-watch or slightly larger, in the middle of which is a button that can be pressed if an emergency occurs. They are usually linked to the telephone and set in motion an automatic chain of events that will lead to appropriate medical or other assistance being called up. In some parts of the country these are provided free or at a subsidized rental but even if the full cost has to be borne, it is worth it for the peace of mind of all those involved.

Contingency plans should certainly be worked out for the event of your own death; permanent alternative care will be required and your own funeral has to be organized. These are matters that are best discussed with other members of the family and the general practitioner, even though at the time it may seem unnecessary. Some people even take the trouble to make their own funeral arrangements with a local funeral director, letting their relatives, general practitioner or others know the details. It may also be a wise precaution to lodge details of any plans you have made with your solicitor, along with your will and information about any other relevant matters that you think are important.

Should you have done more?

Those of us working closely with people who have dementia and who get to know well those caring for them are often told by carers that they wished they had done more, particularly after the sufferer has died or been admitted to a home or hospital for long-term care. This is very much tied up with the feelings of guilt discussed earlier. Remember that it is easy to be wise after the event. Remember also that it is very unlikely that you really could have done any more than you have, however much it may now seem that you could or should have. As already mentioned, caring for a person with dementia is a matter of compromises and there will always be room for nagging doubts and worries about the past. Even if you have made a mistake, you must remember that you will not be alone in this. Everybody makes mistakes and most people make theirs without having to cope with the very great strains that are involved in looking after someone with dementia.

You may find that you can help other carers by passing on your experiences, but it may well take a while after bereavement before this is possible. Similarly, some carers who have agreed to allow the sufferer to go into long-term care may feel too guilty to want to go on sharing their experiences with others. Nevertheless it is worth bearing this in mind and continuing to attend the support group or joining one if you are not already a member. Local voluntary organizations such as the nearest branch of the Alzheimer's Disease Society may also be very pleased to have your help in any one of a number of ways.

Whatever happens, try not to let worries about the past prevent you from starting again with your life, and remember that looking after someone with dementia is in itself a major achievement.

A strategy for caring for yourself

Probably the most important thing that you can do is to share your problems. This means not only the physically demanding tasks that are thrust upon you and with which others may be able to help, but also your own emotional responses. Remember that if they are turned inwards they can be very destructive and that it is not until you appreciate that they are a natural response to the predicament you are in that you will be able to come to terms with them.

The next most important thing is to make time for yourself. You are still you. Make use of whatever resources are available to enable you to have some time with family and friends, to go out and enjoy yourself occasionally, and to keep up a pastime or two. Keeping your batteries charged will enable you to cope more effectively and probably for longer, so that the person you are looking after will benefit in the long run as much as you. If you need longer or more regular breaks, it is important to explore not only day-care and sitting-in services, but also whatever forms of intermittent relief are available in your district. Your general practitioner should be able to help with this. It is very important that you do not allow yourself to become isolated.

Plan ahead for problems that may well not occur, but which could crop up, including your own illness and even death. If the worst happens and you become indisposed, at least you won't have to worry quite so much because you will know that matters should be in hand. Most importantly, do take your own health seriously. Ensure that you have regular check-ups for any health problems that already exist and that you report any new symptoms or worries to your general practitioner as early as possible.

Try to accept support from others even if you don't want to trouble your relatives and friends. Many of them will wish to help you and may in their own turn feel rejected if you keep them away.

You need to identify your own warning signals. Most people will come to realize how much they can take without reaching their own breaking-point. Try to ensure that you take some action if you feel things are getting this bad, in order to avoid a crisis situation.

If you find your relationships with friends and family deteriorating, don't blame them or yourself, but try to think carefully about what is going on and discuss the problem with them. They too may need help in understanding what is really at the root of the breakdown in your relationship. Remember that 'united you stand, divided you fall' and that this has a bearing not only on those directly involved but also on the person being cared for.

Take advice and seek support about the changing role that you will most certainly find yourself in.

Remember also that you are probably the single most important person in the life of the sufferer and without you, he or she may well be lost. It is therefore not only for your own benefit that you must try to look after yourself.

11

Nursing

As their dementia progresses many sufferers will develop physical problems. These might range from incontinence and matters of personal hygiene in a person who is still reasonably independent, to the development of pressure sores in a person who is very dependent. The district nurse and other community services can offer a lot of support for problems like these, in terms of prevention as well as treatment. Adopting a positive approach and seeking advice will often considerably lessen the carer's load.

Dressing and personal appearance

Difficulties with dressing fall into two basic categories. The first involves the selection of the right clothes and the second the ability to put them on properly. Selection of appropriate combinations may be helped by keeping clothes together in sets. This means hanging together the trousers, jackets, pullovers, shirts, etc., that go together. As the confusion progresses it will be necessary to lay out the clothes in the correct order, and having a clear idea in your own mind of what goes with what is helpful. Similarly, keeping clothes together in sets will avoid the need to hunt around for articles in different places. It will also be easier for a confused person if clothes that are inappropriate – summer wear during winter, for example – are stored separately.

Most people with dementia eventually have difficulty with

buttons, shoe-laces, buckles, zips, and so on. A careful adaptation of existing clothes or buying new ones to avoid the need for these relatively complicated dressing manoeuvres will help maintain independence a little longer. Buttons can often be replaced with Velcro tape, but in the later stages it may be best to avoid, as much as possible, clothes that are a potential problem.

Remember also to avoid materials that need dry cleaning. Clothes tend to get dirtier when the person wearing them is muddled and not only is dry cleaning expensive but it is also inconvenient. Bear in mind that many modern fabrics don't need ironing.

Personal appearance is much affected by hairstyling and, for women in particular, by make-up. There are many short, attractive hairstyles for women that are easy to manage; most men prefer their hair cut relatively short in any case. Many of my patients' relatives have arranged for a hairdresser to cut the sufferer's hair in his or her own home. There are more mobile women's hairdressers than there are men's, but most women hairdressers will also be prepared to cut a man's hair.

Hair-washing can be a problem. If it is difficult to manage this during a routine bath or shower, then sitting the person concerned on a chair in front of the kitchen sink or bathroom basin, if big enough, may make for a less physically demanding task. A shower attachment, even if it is not a permanent fixture, is a great help.

It is very important not to forget the need to cut toenails. Fingernails are usually not forgotten and are relatively easy for the carer to manage. If toenails are a problem – and they are often hard and horny in older people – it may be better to arrange for a regular visit to or from a chiropodist. In many parts of the country this is not as simple as it sounds as there is a shortage of trained chiropodists. If this is the case in your own area, you may well find that the district nurse will undertake this task for you.

For many husbands, helping a confused wife apply make-up

seems a waste of time. This is by no means always the case, particularly early on in the course of a dementing illness. The application of even simple make-up such as face powder and lipstick often seems to have a positive effect, although sometimes it is difficult to define quite what this is. It may have an effect on the manner in which other people, even the husband himself, relate to the sufferer. Many people with dementia are still capable of responding to encouragement and this includes positive comments about their appearance.

Personal hygiene

The first requirement is the need to change dirty or soiled clothes regularly, and the second, washing and bathing. Some of the problems surrounding dressing have already been referred to, but the most difficult situation is a confused person who refuses to change his or her clothes. This usually happens when the suggestion is made after the person has already dressed and is most easily overcome by arranging for the provision of clean clothes and the removal of dirty ones either last thing at night or first thing in the morning.

Having a bath or a shower can also be a problem and if it provokes a catastrophic reaction it may be better to accept that there will be fewer baths if a daily routine can't be established. Do remember to make sure that someone checks the temperature of the bath water. A bedbath, although sometimes successful, is often more problematic than an ordinary bath.

It is particularly important to ensure that the skin areas around the genitalia, the patient's bottom, and the areas in skin folds, including under a woman's breasts, are thoroughly attended to. If this is not scrupulously done, superficial skin infections will take a hold, with resulting discomfort and unpleasant odours. To prevent the skin becoming chafed and sore, ensure that it is completely dry after washing or bathing. Follow towelling with talcum powder, especially in areas under skin folds.

Safety in the bathroom is paramount. As well as non-slip mats and rails in the bath and shower, make sure that the floor will not become slippery if water is spilt on it, as is the case with linoleum. Modern bathroom carpeting is very effective, but expensive. An alternative, although second best, is a substantial bath-mat fixed firmly in place with Velcro pads, attached both to the linoleum and the underneath of the mat.

Many people believe a shower to be more unsafe than the bath. This need not be so, as many baths have high sides and it is when negotiating these that accidents happen. A shower cubicle with a chair or stool within it and a shower head attached to a flexible hose is often easier for a relative or other carer to manage.

Using the toilet

As a demented person becomes less steady on his or her feet, it is essential to ensure that rails are provided around the toilet area. Most falls occur when a person is in the process of standing up or sitting down; it is possible to get raised toilet seats that make it easier to get on and off.

For night-time use it may be better to have a commode put at the bedside. This is particularly useful if the bathroom is on a different floor to the bedroom. For men, a bottle-urinal may be helpful not only at night, but also during the day. It can be discreetly placed in a container at the side of the chair in which he is sitting, and regularly emptied.

When a man with dementia begins to forget to go to the bathroom and when, having got there, he has difficulty in remembering the routine, it may be easier for him to sit on the toilet to pass water than to stand up. This can be less problematical and less embarrassing for a wife or other carers.

Problems with using the bathroom and toilet, and many others such as dressing, are an area where the occupational therapist can give invaluable support and advice. This can usually be arranged through the general practitioner or health visitor.

Incontinence

Nearly all those suffering from a dementing illness will eventually lose control of their bowels and their bladder. When this problem first arises, with bed- or seat-wetting, it is essential that it is brought to the attention of the general practitioner as there are many causes of incontinence apart from dementia that older people in particular are prone to. These range from urinary tract infections, such as cystitis, to more important physical problems, such as an enlarged prostate gland, which can be rectified. Although incontinence is most likely to be the result of dementia, it may not be, and this possibility needs to be carefully examined.

It is also important to differentiate between incontinence, which is the inadvertent passage of urine or faeces, and inappropriate behaviour, such as evacuating the bowel or the bladder into the wastepaper basket or the sink. The latter is a behavioural problem rather than true incontinence and can often be helped by making access to a toilet easier or by taking the person concerned to the toilet frequently, so that they don't have to try and find the toilet urgently when they are on their own.

Some people become incontinent because they can't get to the bathroom quickly enough. Again, this is sometimes caused or aggravated by medical conditions which the doctor may be able to treat. If not, easy access to the bathroom and frequent visits to it may also avoid accidents, as described above. At night, leaving a light on, clearly labelling the bathroom door, or providing a chamber pot or commode may be helpful.

It is impossible for a person to be incontinent of urine if the bladder is empty. The need to pass urine is often regulated by the pattern of intake of fluid – drinking habits and mealtime routines – and also sometimes the medication that a person is taking. By carefully charting the times when an incontinent person goes to the bathroom and those when he or she is wet, it may be possible to establish when and how frequently the bladder will need to be emptied. This pattern can then be used to indicate the most appropriate times to take the sufferer to the bathroom to try to avoid a full bladder and consequent incontinence.

Incontinence at night can sometimes be limited by restricting the amount of fluid that is available during the evening. Most people can manage as long as fluid is unrestricted during the remainder of the day. Before adopting this routine, however, it is probably best to check with the sufferer's doctor.

There are also many non-verbal clues that indicate when people need to empty their bladder. The most obvious of course is restlessness, but men may begin to fiddle with their clothing or women to raise their skirts. Keeping a look-out for such signs is often helpful.

Inability to control bowel function can also be caused by medical problems, some of which can be rectified quite easily. Most common of these is severe constipation, with a 'paradoxical' leakage of fluid bowel contents to the outside, rather as if the bowel is overflowing. If, however, the incontinence is the result not of a medical problem, but rather of the dementing process, it can be more difficult to manage. Nevertheless it can be managed even if it can't always be prevented. Sometimes it is necessary to use a combination of different medicines to prevent the bowel being emptied when this would be inappropriate, but on the other hand to stimulate a bowel movement at a convenient time.

A simpler approach which works in some people is to rely upon what is known as the *gastro-colic reflex*. If the stomach is distended by a large quantity of food or fluid this sometimes causes contraction in the large bowel, the colon, resulting in a bowel movement. This is why many people have a normal daily routine which involves emptying their bowels after a particular meal. If a person with Alzheimer's disease or a similar condition is given a reasonable-sized breakfast with at least one large mug of tea, this may well be sufficient to stimulate the evacuation of the large bowel shortly afterwards. The timing varies from person to person, but in some people it is possible to use this natural reflex to help control bowel function.

Unfortunately many people will continue to lose control both of their bowels and of their bladder, despite the best care and attention of their medical attendants and those looking after them. Under these circumstances it is important to try to minimize the workload that this causes and also to try to make sure that the sufferer's skin is kept as clean and dry as possible. There are many varieties of incontinence pants, pads and nappies that can be used in different combinations to try to protect outer garments, chairs and beds. The best are generally those that soak up any moisture in such a way that it is not in contact with the skin for very long.

In many parts of the country, the community services will provide these aids and so an inquiry, probably first of the district nurse or the health visitor, will let you know what is available locally. It is also possible to obtain protective sheets and pads that prevent urine soaking into a chair or a bed if other means of containing it are unsatisfactory. If there is an incontinence laundry service in your area this will be a major boon. They will regularly take away bed-linen and launder it. Unfortunately this service isn't available in all areas. If laundering linen proves to be a major problem, ask your district nurse to advise you about locally available alternatives, which will often consist of a combination of disposable pads and special draw-sheets to protect the bed.

There are many types of urinal that can be strapped on to the man's penis to collect his urine. Some of these are quite effective in the daytime but in general they are not much help at night as they tend to leak. There are no satisfactory appliances of this type for women. For this reason, many medical or paramedical professionals may consider the use of a catheter. This should be avoided if at all possible, but in the last instance it may be necessary. If it makes the difference between a person being able to stay in her own home or having to live in an institution, it is probably better to accept a catheter. It is not necessary for anybody other than the patient and her carers to know that this decision has been taken as the bag into which the catheter drains can be discreetly strapped to a thigh or suspended from a belt within the outer clothing. It is very easy to empty a catheter bag, but necessary to remember that this task should be undertaken as carefully as possible to avoid introducing bacteria into the system.

Nutritional problems

Everyone needs to eat a well-balanced and nutritious diet. This is particularly important as a person gets older because the body is not quite so good at utilizing the essential foodstuffs as it was earlier in life. Many relatives become worried because the person they are looking after becomes less interested in food and may not eat at all on occasions. Another problem concerns the time that meals take to prepare. It often seems easier to use convenience foods if all the other problems caused by dementia make major inroads into the time available for the daily routine.

In most parts of the country, meals-on-wheels are available at least once or twice a week and although there is no choice of menu, or if so it is very restricted, the food is usually nutritious and the meal well-balanced. This is important for both the carer and the sufferer. There are also luncheon clubs but these are often difficult to get to, particularly if you feel you can't take the dementia sufferer there. In many communities, even small villages, local pubs will often be prepared to provide meals that can be taken away. In some communities they will even deliver them regularly to an elderly confused person living on his or her own. This tends to be more expensive than meals-on-wheels, but is nevertheless a good investment.

Neighbours can be a great help in circumstances like this, for if a meal is being prepared for four people it is not really a very much greater task to increase the ingredients to feed six. This may be considerably less expensive than buying in food from a pub, local restaurant or take-away service. Keep convenience foods, whether dried, tinned, or frozen, as a back-up rather than as a mainstay of your diet.

If you are worried about the diet that you and your confused relative may be eating seek advice from the health visitor attached to your local general practice. Prevention of illness, including that resulting from a poor diet, is one of their major functions.

Try and make mealtimes part of the regular daily routine. Don't experiment too much with new dishes but rely upon the familiar. Don't worry if the sufferer appears not to be eating, unless you think he or she is losing weight. We can manage with much less food than we often realize. In the later stages of the disease, failure to eat may be caused by an inability to remember how to eat. It is at this point in the illness that it is necessary to spoon-feed the sufferer. Always make sure that solid food is cut into small pieces as it may not necessarily be chewed properly. If food intake really begins to decline and there is no obvious reason for this, such as a sore mouth or difficulty with swallowing (which should be referred to the doctor), a diet can be boosted with Complan or similar dietary supplements. The problem with some of these, if given in large quantities, is that they can cause diarrhoea. Whenever possible they should be used as a dietary supplement rather than an alternative to normal food. If a full meal is never eaten, substitute instead small regular meals more frequently.

It is very important to remember that if a person stops eating, it may be because he or she has a painful mouth. Ill-fitting dentures are probably the most common cause of this and more and more dentists are beginning to realize that people with dementia have particular problems. If at any time there seems to be any suggestion of discomfort within the mouth, ask your dentist for an appointment. If it is difficult to take the sufferer to the dentist, many dentists will make a home visit to assess the situation.

Nowadays more and more old people have retained some teeth, even if they also wear dentures. They can of course suffer from the same dental problems that the rest of us are subject to, and regular dental inspections are essential. Dentures should be cleaned at least once a day, if not after every meal. Do remember that ill-fitting dentures cause sores in the mouth which may not be visible unless carefully looked for, and that these in turn may lead to a person with dementia refusing to eat.

Pressure sores

Pressure sores used to be called bed sores because they were associated with a person lying for long periods in one position, in bed. As they also occur under other circumstances, for instance when a person is sitting for a prolonged period in a chair, and the factor common to the development of this type of sore is prolonged pressure, they have been renamed. This is more important than it may at first appear as it reminds one that prolonged pressure, of any kind, may result in the breakdown of the skin wherever this pressure is applied.

Areas that are particularly vulnerable are those sites on the body where skin is fairly close to bony projections and this includes the heels, the ankles, the buttocks and the spine. Often the first indication that an area of skin is at risk of breaking down is a slight redness. The skin in older people is more fragile than in many younger people and this fragility is aggravated by inadequate nutrition and prolonged contact with moisture, perhaps occurring because of urinary incontinence. In the later stages of a dementing illness sufferers are often relatively immobile, even if they can still walk a little and are not necessarily in a bed or sitting on a chair all the time.

Prevention is always better than cure. Relatively immobile people should be encouraged to get up and do something simple from time to time and not stay in the same position for more than an hour or so at a stretch. In theory a bed-bound person should be turned at least every two hours, but this is often not possible in the home environment and other means have to be used to take pressure off the danger areas, as described below. In particular, try to make sure that the confused person never sits with his or her legs crossed all the time, particularly if the outside of one ankle is resting against the same area on the other.

There are many aids to prevent pressure sores developing, and these range from a simple sheepskin (or synthetic equivalent) for the seat of a chair or fashioned into the form of heel-protectors, to more complicated cushions or mattresses divided up into a large number of air-filled cells which inflate and deflate automatically, varying the points of the body that are subject to pressure. The local district nurse is usually an expert at prevention, as well as being skilled in the treatment of existing sores.

Infections

A debilitated person, one suffering from a chronic disease, is more likely to suffer from infections. Some of these have already been mentioned, such as the skin rashes that develop in hot sweaty places that are not kept clean and the infection that can occur in the urinary tract, causing cystitis and frequently incontinence of urine. There are many other infections, the most important of which is probably pneumonia. There may well be little outward sign of pneumonia because many old people don't have a rise in temperature or produce phlegm as younger people do when they develop the infection. It can only be diagnosed by a doctor's careful examination. Often the only clue to the presence of any infection may be a worsening of the level of confusion. If this happens without there being an obvious cause, it is important to ask the doctor to come and assess the situation.

Constipation

Constipation is a very common problem in older people. Because so many people with dementia are old, many of them also suffer in this way. As mentioned in the section on incontinence, severe constipation can actually cause a form of faecal incontinence and if severe enough it can, strangely, sometimes lead to incontinence of urine as well. Many people only empty their bowels every three or four days and if this has been their normal routine, there is no point in trying to persuade them to empty their bowels more frequently. If, however, as for most people, this has been a daily routine, it doesn't really matter if it becomes a little less frequent, such as every alternate day. This is particularly true if the person concerned is eating significantly less than he or she used to.

One of the best ways of keeping bowels functioning normally is to ensure that there is an adequate amount of roughage, or fibre, in the diet. This helps the bowels to move the food along from one end of the alimentary tract to the other. A diet that is high in convenience foods, sweets and cake is unlikely to contain an adequate amount of fibre. Wholemeal bread, cereals containing bran and fresh fruit and vegetables are amongst the most palatable forms of fibre.

Some people have used purgatives all their lives and under these circumstances constipation can be very difficult to cure, adequate fibre intake on its own being insufficient to restore normal bowel function. If there is a problem, the doctor and the district nurse can usually assess its severity and recommend treatment.

Pain

Sometimes when there is something wrong with people with dementia all that they can indicate to us is that they are in discomfort. This may be apparent from an increased level of agitation or a deterioration in their behavioural pattern. It can be extremely difficult to discover whether pain really is the cause of increased confusion and, if so, what it is caused by. The source of pain can be a full bladder that won't empty, as happens in some men with an enlarged prostate gland, or perhaps an undetected broken bone; indigestion from ulcers can also be the culprit, and so on. A person with dementia is just as likely to develop all the physical problems that the rest of us can have. All that the doctor can normally do is exclude obvious and easily diagnosed causes of pain, and if a specific diagnosis is not apparent, treat the pain in a general way in the hope either that it will settle down or that other indicators of the underlying problem will eventually become apparent.

Convulsions

Convulsions, which are sometimes known as fits, seizures or epilepsy, can be very frightening. They do occur in a small number of people with dementia, but not in the majority. Again, like so many other symptoms, they can be caused by illnesses other than the dementia and so it is important that a doctor establishes that there is no other cause that might be treatable.

Most fits can, in fact, be prevented by medicines, so if convulsions become a major problem, the frequency with which they occur can be considerably reduced and often they can be prevented altogether.

Fits are usually associated with loss of consciousness, jerking movements of the arms and legs, and sometimes the whole body and the head and neck, disturbance of breathing pattern, and in some a period of extreme stiffness. This is the picture of a full-blown fit, but very often they are much less dramatic, involving only abnormal movements of a single limb for a short period. The disturbed electrical activity may, however, affect the whole brain and this can result in a period of sleepiness or drowsiness after the fit is over.

Although they can be alarming to onlookers, fits rarely result in any harm to the sufferer. When they do, the damage is usually caused by trauma resulting from the abnormal movements, or a head injury if the fit is accompanied by a fall. Sometimes a person vomits while they are fitting, or shortly afterwards. For this reason it is best to lay those who have had a fit on their side or face downwards, but making sure that they can still breathe and that their breathing passages are not obstructed. The ideal position is that known to first-aid workers as 'semiprone'.

The side-effects of medication

If a change occurs in the behaviour of people with dementia or they seem otherwise to be behaving abnormally, it is important to consider whether or not the change is the result of a side-effect of any medication that is being prescribed. Older people are much more sensitive to unwanted effects of prescribed medicines and also those that you can buy over the counter without a prescription. Prescriptions ought not to be repeated indefinitely, every month say, without a formal review taking place from time to time. The frequency of the review will depend to a certain extent on the problems being treated and the nature of the drugs being prescribed. Many older people, even those not suffering with a dementing illness, can be prescribed a medicine for a particular problem and then three years later it is discovered that they are still taking the same drugs even though the problem may have receded long ago.

Every so often, people with dementia may refuse to take their pills. If a medicine is being taken two or three times a day, it probably doesn't matter very much if an occasional dose is omitted. This is best checked with the doctor who prescribed the pills as there are some exceptions. If refusal to take medication is a consistent and protracted problem, it may be necessary to ask the doctor to prescribe an alternative form of the drug, for example a liquid that can be mixed with a cold drink or a capsule containing a powder such that the capsule can be opened and the powder mixed with jam, honey, or something else that is palatable.

It is better to always assume that a person who is confused and forgetful will need to have his or her drug-taking supervised. In the early stages, if this is impossible, there are various tricks that may help to ensure that medication is taken properly. Some drugs come in calendar packs and if not, it is possible to buy a similar gadget, such as a plastic box divided up into compartments, each labelled with the day of the week. In some such boxes the compartments are further divided into three or four subsections so that the medicines for morning, noon, and night can be placed in their own compartment. This is helpful to those supervising the medicines as it may give an indication of how frequently the pills are being forgotten.

Finally, there are three types of side-effect that commonly occur when a medicine is given to try to control abnormal or difficult behaviour in a person with dementia, and which you should look out for. These are: difficulty in walking – a tendency to fall or stumble, especially after rising from a chair or getting out of bed; increased sedation, i.e. sleepiness in the daytime; and restlessness.

Choosing a nursing home

Many of the physical and behavioural problems that occur during a dementing illness make it impossible for a member of the family to carry on caring right up until the end. Under these circumstances some sufferers will be admitted for long-term care, e.g. to a nursing home or a residential home for the elderly mentally infirm. 'Quality control' of the care that your relative receives will have to be mainly your responsibility.

Many nursing homes won't wish to take on people with dementia, for various reasons, and the fees for those that will may seem very high. The same is often true for private residential homes. Nevertheless there are a number of statutory grants that are available, some of which are means-tested, to help families meet the costs of such care. The social worker attached to your local general practice or to the hospital – if the sufferer is attending as an in-patient or day-patient – will be able to give advice on sources of funding and provide you with a list of nursing homes. It is unlikely that social workers will be prepared to recommend one against another, and this is only fair, as different aspects of different homes will appeal to different people.

Before making the decision that you can no longer cope, do make sure that all possible community resources have been made available to you. Many carers are unaware of the support that they can call upon locally. Many of these services have been described elsewhere, but it is important to realize that even if available in theory, some of them may be very thin on the ground, especially as the number of older people with dementia is rapidly increasing.

Making a decision like this is very much a matter for the family and it is important to discuss it with the other relatives who are involved. You can also take professional advice from the general practitioner, or a member of his or her team, or from an appropriate member of the hospital staff if your relative is a hospital patient.

The difference between nursing homes and residential homes needs to be stressed. In the latter, whether provided by the social services, a voluntary body, or privately run, nursing care is not usually available. Each resident has to be fairly independent and more than a minor degree of confusion is unacceptable unless it is a home specifically for the elderly mentally infirm.

Some homes are dual registered, which means that they can take reasonably independent people in the early stages of an illness and continue to care for them when they need the sort of help that is usually only available in a nursing home.

All homes are overseen by either the local authority or the

health service, at least in principle. The degree of supervision, however, varies significantly from region to region.

It is very difficult to know which home is most appropriate for a particular individual. What seems best for one person may not suit another at all. Close relatives and carers are often best placed to make this decision, as they will often get a 'feel' for the home and for how their relative will fit in there. Don't accept a place simply because it is the first empty bed that you come across. Visit a number of homes, ask to see around, and inquire about the points listed at the end of this section, as well as any other matters that you think are particularly important.

As you go round the home, try to establish whether it feels homely, whether the residents are sitting around doing nothing; if you see a member of staff talking to or helping a resident, try to assess their attitude. It is also important to look carefully in the bathroom areas for adequate safety features such as rails and non-slip surfaces. Also make sure that it is clean. Above all, try to imagine how happy your relative would be there.

Ask whether it is possible for your relative to be admitted for a fortnight or so in the first instance to see how he or she gets on. This will give everyone an opportunity to assess at first hand how things will go. If a sudden transition is likely to cause a major degree of upset, some homes will allow potential residents to attend on a daily basis several times a week, rather like going to a day centre or a day hospital. This manoeuvre can sometimes be used to ease a person with dementia from one environment to another.

Finally, beware of brochures. These can be very helpful, but they can also be extremely misleading. It is better to use your own eyes, to listen carefully, and to try to pick up the general atmosphere. No matter how splendid the surroundings and the fitments may appear to be, don't forget that the most important aspect of a nursing home is probably the attitude of the staff, both to those that they are looking after and also to their relatives.

Points to consider when choosing a nursing home
- Are rooms shared or single?
- Are personal possessions and furniture allowed?
- What are the visiting arrangements?
- What activities are encouraged, other than watching the television?
- What is the menu for a typical week?
- Can residents keep their existing general practitioner?
- How many trained nursing staff are available during the day and at night?
- Have they ever had to ask residents to leave – if so why?
- Do residents have their own washing and toilet facilities?
- How large are the bedrooms and sitting rooms?
- Is there the aroma of urine?
- How flexible is the daily routine, e.g. mealtimes?

Care in a residential home

Much of what has been said about nursing homes is relevant also to residential home care. Many people with dementia who live on their own may well need to go into residential care when they can no longer be maintained in their own home, despite the fullest use of community services. This will often happen well before the stage at which they need nursing care, and the choice will usually be between the social services welfare home, or 'Part III accommodation', and a private residential home. The local authority will levy a charge on the demented person's estate, after applying a means-test, if he or she has any financial resources. Private residential home charges are often higher than those in local authority homes, but there are many statutory grants that will help cover the cost.

Most residential homes cannot cope with a heavy, physical nursing load nor with markedly impaired behaviour unless the home is specifically designed for this type of resident. It is very likely therefore that the time will come when a demented person in a residential home will have to move on to alternative accommodation, most usually a nursing home. This of course is where the dual registered homes come in.

The criteria for choosing an appropriate residential home

Private residential homes are often smaller and more homely than local authority homes, but this is by no means always the case. Staffing levels may vary considerably between homes and although it is not so important to have trained nursing staff to hand, it is essential to inquire about the staffing ratios and the qualifications of those employed.

Arranging for a confused relative to be admitted to a home can seem a major problem. The person to help you most is the social worker. He or she should get to know your relative, provide you with a list of homes, point out the sorts of things you ought to be taking into consideration, beyond those mentioned in this book, and help you with the financial arrangements. The social worker should also be able to assist you with any worries and reservations you may have about placing your relative in a home, and may be prepared to keep in touch with you for a while afterwards, as the emotions that are sometimes aroused by such a move can be very distressing for the carers who have arranged it.

It may be more difficult to persuade a person early on in the course of his or her illness to enter a residential home than to persuade a more demented elderly person to accept a move to a nursing home. It is important that you, and if necessary also the social worker concerned, try to involve your relative in making this decision. Again, gradual habituation to the new environment by occasional day attendance may make it easier. Because many residential homes are unhappy about taking on very confused people, occasional attendance of this sort will give them the opportunity of assessing whether or not they think they can cope. It will also give you the opportunity to assess how they react to your relative and to assist in making the decision as to whether or not placement in a nursing home may be more appropriate.

Dying

Once a person's dementia has progressed beyond a certain stage, the duration of life becomes less important than its quality. Most people, be they family carers or professional advisors, would not wish to preserve at all costs an existence that might be a burden to the sufferer. A discussion between the family and the doctors will usually result in a joint decision about the most appropriate form of treatment. In some circumstances treatment may need to be fairly active, but in others it may consist merely in ensuring that the person with dementia does not suffer pain, distress or thirst. It is the doctors' and nurses' job to try to help people die with dignity and with the least suffering possible.

Sometimes, a demented person's illness, a pneumonia for example, may look certain to end in his or her death and it will be decided not to treat the infection, but rather to pay attention to alleviating distress and suffering. After a few days, however, it may become apparent that despite not being treated with antibiotics, the patient is rallying and the pneumonia receding. Under these circumstances many doctors will elect to institute treatment with antibiotics to speed up the recovery, rather than allow it to take place over a prolonged period of time resulting eventually in a greater degree of dependence and a lessened quality of life than would otherwise have been the case. The point at which to intervene with antibiotics in such cases is often difficult to determine and it is not possible to lay ground rules. Each situation has to be considered on its own merits.

Few, if any, people die of dementia, the majority succumbing to intercurrent infections such as pneumonia. Sometimes, however, other factors contribute to a patient's death, for example malnutrition and a failure to drink. The body in general will deteriorate, sometimes slowly, sometimes not so slowly, until the sufferer dies. The exact mechanism of this is often uncertain as it can appear to occur without a specific intercurrent illness.

As discussed in an earlier chapter, when a person with dementia does die, it is possible that the doctors may ask whether you would be prepared to give permission for a post-mortem examination of the brain. Many relatives find this a difficult decision to make, often because they haven't been given the opportunity to think about it in advance. Often the only definite way of making a diagnosis of the condition that has caused the dementia is to examine the brain after death. It is extremely helpful to doctors to have their suspicions about the diagnosis confirmed, or the reverse. Knowledge gained in this way may well help them in the management of their future patients.

We also need to know a lot more about the changes that occur in the brain in people who have dementia and much of the research can only be undertaken on brain tissue donated at a post-mortem examination. The new approaches to treatment and increased understanding that we have recently gained have nearly all been based upon the results of research carried out using post-mortem material. There is no reason why a post-mortem examination should significantly delay the arrangements for a funeral and it will not cause any further suffering to the deceased. The examination is undertaken in a very discreet manner and there is usually little, if any, evidence that it has taken place.

In many cases it is very likely that if the deceased sufferer had appreciated in earlier life what sort of illness he or she was going to develop, he or she would have given permission in advance for a post-mortem examination, in the hope that it might contribute knowledge that might help doctors and medical scientists to treat others.

12

Preserving Independence

Although in the course of most forms of dementia the time will arrive when sufferers will become less involved with their environment and those around them because of apathy, loss of concentration, and so on, it is best to make the most of what they can achieve while this is still possible. Life will then become fuller not just for the sufferer, but also for those who are involved in caring. This chapter describes some simple activities that may be possible in the early and mid stages of the disease. Rather than trying to keep a person with dementia active all day long, it is probably better to break up the day by organizing several short periods of activity at convenient times. In the earlier stages of the disease it may be helpful to concentrate upon those that will result in the sufferer enjoying a feeling of achievement and having been useful.

Other important areas that relate to the preservation of independence are the need to stop driving, to give up work, to give up living alone, and often to move house. These will all be discussed in turn.

It is not usually possible for people with dementia to easily learn new skills so it is best to base activities, whether recreational or otherwise, on skills that have already been obtained in earlier life, taking advantage of them until they fade from the memory store. Activities that involve relationships with other people and pets are often among the most meaningful for a person with a declining intellect. It is also important to remember the need for physical exercise.

This chapter will only be able to provide ideas, as with so many of the other chapters in this book. Trial and error alone will show what is best for an individual and his or her pattern of activity should not be expected to remain unchanged as the months pass.

Reminiscence

Many older people like to think back over their lives and this can give great pleasure. One of the assets that a dementia sufferer usually has are his or her early memories. This ability is sometimes used therapeutically in day hospitals and other settings, for example encouraging people with dementia to draw pictures of their past, use photographs and other visual material to make a collage, or write notes if this is still possible. A folder of relevant material or a box of objects relating to the past can be used many times in an attempt to bring out happy memories. Old photographs of family, friends, holidays, weddings, and so on are also helpful. Records, or somebody playing music from the past on the piano, will often evoke memories that may stimulate conversation.

An alternative approach is to use stimuli, such as pictures or music, as part of a simple game. Often the questions can be made up as one goes along and a single object can be used repeatedly as the basis for different questions.

Household tasks

Many household tasks can be broken up into simple, step-by-step instructions. Cooking is a favourite activity in many day hospitals and day centres because it is not too complex, does not involve much walking around, and people often have a feeling of satisfaction when they can see what they have achieved, and also eat it. It must be remembered, however, that we often make conceptual jumps in our own minds when we perform such tasks. A simple instruction such as 'add two tablespoons of sugar to the mixture' will often be insufficient for people with dementia. The time will come when they may also have to be told where the sugar is, which spoon to use, and to be reminded what the word 'two' means. For this reason it is important to concentrate on the simplest of recipes. Those that don't take long to cook are the best as they may be ready to come out of the oven or off the stove as part of a continuous process that sufferers can relate to what has gone before; for they may not remember that a cake that has been taken out of the oven has anything to do with their having put the ingredients together two hours earlier.

Many other household activities can also be broken down into simple steps, such that a spouse or other carer can supervise at the same time as doing something else.

It is also often very rewarding for both the person with dementia and the carer if some simple activities can be undertaken together, such that each is an equal partner in the activity, for example wiping and drying the dishes, hanging washing on the line or bringing it in, and folding it up and putting it away after the ironing has been completed. It is much more satisfying for a person with dementia if it is something they can undertake without feeling they are being instructed or organized. Don't therefore worry too much if the outcome isn't perfect and try to avoid being critical. Finally, it is important not to forget to express appreciation and thanks even if, in reality, their involvement has not made the task any easier! Remember to laugh if things go wrong as this will diffuse what might otherwise become an awkward situation.

Gardening

Many people have enjoyed gardening during their life and will retain certain basic skills, physical problems permitting. A small piece of garden in which simple flowers or vegetables can be grown may provide a lot of stimulation. As well as the need to plant and sow and then to tend the growing plants, it can be an interesting focus of attention on other occasions. A short stroll into the garden, especially if it is sunny, can be very soothing. It can also be used as a diversional activity to be returned to at times of stress or agitation.

If an outdoor plot is, or becomes, impractical for any reason, consider creating an indoor garden with plants in pots or trays on the windowsill, in a conservatory, or elsewhere. It is best to use unbreakable or inexpensive materials and to grow simple plants. These could be purely decorative, grown only for interest, or productive such as mustard and cress, beansprouts, and even indoor tomatoes if the space allows.

Exercise

Exercise is very important, not only for a person with dementia but also for yourself. If you are the main carer for a person with dementia you may very well have to take exercise together. Not only does this help with physical well-being, but it also has a beneficial effect on the mind, relieving tension and promoting psychological health.

Without doubt the easiest form of exercise for older people, particularly older people with dementia, is walking. This needn't necessarily be a gentle amble, pleasant though this can be, but a brisk stroll. If physical disabilities allow, walking briskly for about half an hour, sufficient to raise the pulse rate a little and to feel a little hot, will be of constitutional benefit.

Even if it is possible for you to manage it, it is probably best to avoid exercise that leaves you short of breath and perspiring heavily. If you have any doubts about the exercise tolerance of either yourself or the person you are looking after, it is very important to consult your doctor. Exercise needn't be taken every day; two or three times a week is probably enough.

There are many different games that involve exercise, but the physical content of these is less important than the personal interaction that they usually generate with other people. Although they tend to be played in a day centre or a day hospital there is no reason why they can't be practised at home if there are enough people. They can be simple games such as passing a ball around by gently throwing or rolling, or more demanding ones, such as skittles, depending upon the severity of the dementia. It is usually not difficult to devise simple activities of this kind which not only involve a certain amount of physical exercise, a feeling of enjoyment, and social interaction with others, but also result in the participants practising co-ordination.

Some people advocate the sort of physical exercises that young people used to do in gymnastic classes – stretching, bending, jumping, and so on. In my experience these don't very often appeal to people with dementia and it is also important to stop them falling off-balance. Nevertheless they may be appropriate for some dementia sufferers.

Music

There is no reason at all why a person with dementia can't enjoy music. Sitting and listening passively will give pleasure to many, as will taking a more active role, such as joining in by humming or singing. More importantly, those who have learnt to play a musical instrument in earlier life may retain this skill, at a simple level, much further into the course of the disease than one would expect. This can give great pleasure and a sense of achievement, not only to them, but also to those looking after them.

For listening to music, it is probably better to rely on cassette recorders than record players as the former are easier to switch on and off. There is also little danger of damaging the cassette. If the music would disturb others, it is worth trying a personal cassette player with a pair of headphones, of the sort now widely used.

Even if a musical person loses the skill to play an instrument, but retains some musical abilities, it may be possible to substitute simple home-made instruments such as drums made from cans or rattles created by filling tins or jars with beans.

Handicrafts

Some mention has already been made about creating collages and scrapbooks. In the earlier stages of dementia, activities like these can reasonably be embarked upon. However, the sufferer will need a lot of supervision and tactful help. Take care if dangerous objects such as scissors, tools, nails, and so on are used.

Scrapbooks, collages, mobiles and many other such projects can be the focus of much interest, can help with practising coordination and other intellectual skills, and result in a feeling of achievement. One daughter I know took home many ideas she gained from her work as an infant school teacher and found that her mother with Alzheimer's disease enjoyed most of those that she was able to attempt.

Activities that are undertaken alone

Don't forget that there are many interesting and stimulating activities that do not require continuous supervision. Sensible use of the television is one, particularly if the programmes chosen relate to something that was formerly of interest to the sufferer. Reading, even if this is in reality only looking at pictures, can also provide some interest and stimulation and many of the games that have been developed for young children can be adapted to engage the attention of a person with dementia.

Pets

It has now been convincingly shown that pets, especially those that can be held or stroked, are of major benefit to elderly people. This is almost certainly true for those who have dementia as well. Cats and dogs are the likeliest pets which can sit on one's lap. Take care, however, that they don't cause accidents, such as when a cat winds itself round one's feet. You need not necessarily keep a pet in your own home if neighbours will lend you theirs! Trips to visit an animal can be just as beneficial as having your own.

Driving

Deciding when a person with dementia should no longer drive a car is a very tricky problem. Not only is it usually a matter of pride for the driver, but the ability to get about by car can be of great practical importance in the everyday life of the sufferer and his or her carers. It is therefore very tempting to assume that all is well when there is no obvious risk. Driving is an automatic activity that often doesn't appear to require thought – until some untoward event occurs, that is. It is quite possible for a person with dementia to undertake a journey that he or she has made many times in the past without any difficulty at all. However, should something happen that requires fast and logical thought to avoid an accident, or the road layout be unexpectedly changed, major problems can ensue. Although familiar journeys in the daylight will probably remain possible for some time, as the dementia progresses an attempt to make a journey that breaks new ground may well produce a crisis and, if you are unlucky, an accident. As soon as you are aware that driving ability is even only a little impaired by dementia, it is essential that the person concerned stops driving, but if you are in any doubt, consult your doctor. There is also a legal requirement to inform the licensing authority of any disability that may impair fitness to drive, unless it is only a temporary affliction. Most if not all insurance companies also require their policy holders to be fit to drive. It is technically possible, if an accident were to happen and the insurance company were to argue that the driver responsible was unfit through mental incapacity, that they would consider the insurance invalid. Not only could this result in their failing to make appropriate financial compensation, it might also leave the driver open to a charge of driving without insurance.

It is therefore probably a good idea to start getting a person who has early dementia used to the fact that he or she will eventually have to give up the car. This may well cause great sadness or anger. Nevertheless it will eventually be in the best interests of all concerned.

If you are unable to prevent a relative with dementia from driving by reasoning with him or her, you may have to 'lose' the car keys or, if necessary with the help of a friend, immobilize the car by some means. A belief that it has broken down may act as a natural break-point, enabling you to persuade your relative that it is not worth making the necessary repairs.

This is a situation that must be dealt with gently and tactfully, avoiding confrontation if possible. If you can drive yourself, you may be able to think of an excuse to do the driving on most, if not all, occasions. Remember that being able to drive a car requires physical fitness (good sight and hearing especially), coordination, and the intellectual ability to react and make decisions rapidly when this is necessary. You may find that your doctor will be able to help you if your advice to stop driving goes unheeded.

Giving up work

Many people who develop dementia do so after they have retired, and therefore don't have to contemplate giving up their job. When dementia strikes during working life, the situation can be particularly distressing. What to do about it will depend entirely upon the abilities of the sufferer and the nature of the job. One elderly lady who developed dementia was able to carry on her work as a seamstress until she was seventy by being given increasingly simple tasks by an understanding employer. On the other hand a young person in an extremely demanding and complicated job, such as accountancy, or a person who has to make important management decisions that affect others, may have to resign much earlier. If at all practicable this is a decision that should be made tactfully and sympathetically by the sufferer, the sufferer's family and the employer, taking into account medical advice. Unfortunately it isn't always possible to proceed in this way and very often the employer will approach the next of kin, often feeling guilty and apprehensive, to discuss the need for the sufferer to give up work.

There are many problems surrounding early retirement. It is important to take advice about the financial consequences, as being able to retire at sixty rather than fifty-nine may make an important difference. Sometimes extended sick-leave or a change in the nature of the job may make it possible for retirement to be deferred to a time that would be financially advantageous.

Don't forget that retiring or resigning because of dementia is a matter of ill health, just as if it were the result of a more obvious physical illness.

Living alone

If sufferers are living on their own, the time will probably come when it is no longer safe for them to be allowed to continue as they are. There is a limit to the amount of help that can be provided, unless a friend or relative can be present all the time or somebody can be paid to live in for all or part of the day. The time to move will vary from person to person. It is usually easier to arrange for the confused to have help with dressing, bathing, housework and cooking than it is to prevent them from wandering or being a danger to other people as well as themselves. The risk of accidents is often the final straw for worried relatives. You may decide to allow your relative with dementia to be at risk on his or her own account, but this is neither reasonable nor fair if others may be affected.

Whether or not a person with dementia should continue to

live on his or her own should become a family decision wherever this is possible. The family, of course, includes the sufferer, but sometimes plans have to be made even if not immediately acted upon, without his or her agreement. A family conference can often be helpful and ensures that the responsibility is shared by all. At such meetings families sometimes realize that between them, if they all pull together, it may be possible to prolong the independence of their relative with dementia.

13

Treatment Strategies

In general, treatment strategies fall into three main groups. The first of these is particularly aimed at those who are supporting others who are looking after a person with dementia and in this chapter we will consider the role of support groups and how to set one up from scratch if necessary. The other two strategies cover behavioural approaches and the use of medication.

Over the years there have been many behavioural approaches to treating people with dementia. The best known of these is probably *reality orientation* (RO), but there have been others such as *reminiscence therapy* and *music therapy* that are gaining popularity at the moment. It must be said that their main purpose is to try and maximize whatever intellectual ability remains, rather than improve the situation by resurrecting brain cells or preventing further decline. Many of the commonsense approaches that carers adopt to overcome difficulties are actually reality orientation techniques although not specifically called this. Reality orientation is the application of common sense to provide stimulation and exercise to the failing mental capabilities of a person with Alzheimer's disease or a similar condition.

Reminiscence therapy, music therapy, and similar approaches are, in my opinion, effective methods of improving the quality of life for short periods for many people with dementia. Making the most of long-term memories can bring back pleasurable thoughts and associations, and may sometimes have a calming effect upon the sufferer. Music, particularly that relating to the past, can have a similar effect. When these activities are carried out in a group, it is sometimes possible to stimulate interaction between group members, even when the individuals appear to be quite severely demented. It is, however, often worth trying these or similar approaches in a one-to-one situation if attendance at a group session is not practical.

Behavioural approaches to improving the quality of life of people with dementia are very important, but it often seems as if more is made of their scientific validity than is realistic and this can lead carers and relatives to expect to see an improvement in the intellectual ability of the person they are caring for, after the session or activity is over. This rarely happens; when it does it is usually short-lived and consists most commonly of an elevation of mood.

The therapeutic strategies involving the use of medicines fall into two groups. On the one hand there is the use of existing, well-tried medical approaches to treatment of difficult behaviour in people with dementia. These involve drugs that are well known to most of those looking after a person with dementia, especially professional carers. On the other hand new medicines are being developed and evaluated in the hope that they may slow down, or even reverse, a sufferer's intellectual decline. As mentioned elsewhere, some medicines are now available that help with the symptoms of Alzheimer's disease in some people, albeit mainly to only a modest extent. Although they are technically available within the National Health Service, at the time of writing about half the health authorities in the country are unable to commit funds to support their prescription. Hopefully this will change and medicines like Aricept (Donepezil) and Exelon (Rivastigmine), and those that follow, will become more widely available so that a trial of treatment can be offered to all those in whom it is appropriate, even though long-term administration will probably only be worthwhile in about half of those to whom it is initially prescribed. This is described in greater detail in chapter 4.

Reality orientation

Reality orientation is a technique that is widely applied all over the world where people with dementia are looked after. It is almost impossible to enter a health or social services centre without coming across a large board detailing the day of the week, the month, the day of the month, the year, what the weather is like, and so on. Reality orientation has been well tried now for at least twenty years and is applied not only to people with dementia, but also to others, usually elderly, who for one reason or another have become isolated from their environment.

It is not generally appreciated, even among some professional people, that there are two approaches to reality orientation. *Classroom reality orientation* involves intensive stimulation for periods varying from thirty to sixty minutes a day. Half an hour is usually found to be about as much as most people can tolerate of this intensive stimulation. It involves showing patients information, usually presented on an RO board, sometimes in the form of written information, sometimes using equipment such as clocks, calendars, maps and posters. Tape-slide presentations can also be used and, where appropriate, discussion of simple topics and even role-playing have been tried.

The other form of RO has loosely been called *twenty-four-hour reality orientation*. This usually takes place in a hospital ward or a residential home. Instead of being presented with an intensive information session, the subjects are orientated in their relevant everyday activities throughout the full twenty-four hours. This means, for example, that instead of just telling all the patients that it is now time for supper, or even worse wheeling them into the dining-room without any proper discussion, they are addressed by their name, told the time of day, and informed that it is suppertime and that they will be going to the dining-room – or are asked to make their own way there if they are capable of this. In the case of confused people getting up in the middle of the night and wandering around, rather than just trying to get them back to bed the reality-orientation approach would be to explain to them what is going on, why they shouldn't be wandering around (having tried to ascertain that there wasn't after all a valid reason for this), and generally trying to get them to appreciate why they should go back to bed. This approach is assisted by the very careful and clear labelling of doors, etc., often with a symbol rather than a written word.

Both these approaches have their advocates and it may well be that they are complementary rather than in competition with each other. Nevertheless, in a study where a comparison of the two approaches was made between a group of people who were resident in a psychogeriatric hospital and another group who lived in an old people's home, it was discovered that classroom RO improved brain function a little, but had no effect on behaviour, whereas a highly significant behavioural change was demonstrated for the twenty-four-hour orientation training. The latter also had the advantage of not requiring special apparatus or a trained therapist to organize the sessions.

Finally, a word of caution about behavioural techniques. They are not suitable for all people with dementia and whether or not a particular individual will benefit may well depend upon the stage of his or her disease. Just because it appeared to be beneficial earlier on does not mean that it will always be useful. If attendance at a reality orientation class or attempts to practise twenty-four-hour RO results in distress or aggression, little will be gained. It is important not to impose behavioural training on a person who refuses to co-operate.

The medical treatment of disturbed behaviour

Many different drugs can be used to control disturbed behaviour in a person with dementia. Before any treatment is prescribed, however, it is essential that the doctor and also the others caring for the disturbed person ensure that there isn't an unrelated reason for the behavioural abnormality. One must remember at all times that people with Alzheimer's disease or similar conditions are just as prone to the problems of advancing age as anybody else, if not more so.

A man with a large prostate gland may suddenly find he can't empty his bladder and becomes extremely agitated and aggressive in consequence, and also incontinent. A person with a broken hip may not be able to let you know that he or she is in pain, but may suddenly appear to become obstinate and refuse to get up and walk. People who suddenly become more confused and difficult may have an infection or may even be over-reacting to drugs that they are already taking. In most cases, however, there won't be an obvious underlying contributory factor and a change in behaviour, especially when it involves aggression, wandering in the middle of the night, or something else that is causing distress to others, may well require treatment. Once prescribed this is often continued indefinitely, a frequent mistake. All medication should be considered as a short-term measure, with the medicine slowly discontinued after a period of two or three weeks in the hope that it won't be necessary to re-prescribe it. Even if a further course is eventually necessary, it is better to have infrequent and intermittent courses of medicines than to have them prescribed indefinitely, although sometimes this will be necessary.

All drugs have side-effects and sometimes these can outweigh any benefits. Most of the medicines that are currently prescribed to improve behaviour belong to a group known as the *phenothiazines* or are related to this group. Among the best known are thioridazine, which is also called Melleril, and chlorpromazine, also called Largactil. The latter is best avoided in older people, who tend to be oversensitive to it. There are many different members of this group of drugs but they all have very similar side-effects. Some of these unwanted effects occur more frequently with one drug than another, and some individuals seem more sensitive to one phenothiazine than to another, or particularly prone to develop certain side-effects. All drugs in the phenothiazine group, and other related medicines such as haloperidol, should be avoided in people whose dementia appears to be associated with Lewy bodies. Some people with this condition are particularly prone to the unwanted effects of these drugs and if it is essential to prescribe them, they must be used with great caution and under close medical supervision.

Over-sedation or excessive sleepiness is frequently seen with phenothiazines and can be one of the most difficult and troublesome of the unwanted effects. The difference between the dose required to control the behaviour disturbance and the dose that causes sedation may be very small, so it can be very easy to have a situation where the behaviour is controlled because the subject spends most of the day asleep. This is clearly unsatisfactory and it is sometimes necessary to switch from one form of phenothiazine to another in order to find a preparation that suits an individual sufferer.

There are two side-effects of phenothiazines that affect mobility. The first is known as *postural hypotension* and causes a feeling of dizziness, giddiness, or faintness when, or just after, the person for whom the drug has been prescribed stands up from a sitting or lying position. This leads to unsteadiness and a tendency to fall, and can sometimes be so profound that the sufferer will refuse to get up. It is caused by the drug allowing the blood to collect in the lower parts of the body such that there is insufficient to supply the brain's needs. It is very similar to when a person faints in the heat and indeed people with postural hypotension can sometimes faint, although this occurs infrequently.

The other major problem that interferes with walking is

the development of Parkinsonism, although with Parkinsonism caused by phenothiazines the sufferer does not develop a tremor or shake. What happens instead is that a stiffness of the arms and legs may develop, making it more difficult to move them properly and often resulting in an increased tendency to fall. Probably the most important reason for this is a combination of stiffness and slowness in initiating the natural reflex we all experience when we find ourselves off balance. This happens to all of us many times each day without us realizing it most of the time. Finding oneself off balance for whatever reason is no problem at all if one can rapidly compensate by changing position of part of the trunk or a limb. If one is stiff or, as in the case of Parkinsonism, has a slowness in starting new movements, it is difficult to correct a position of imbalance with the necessary speed.

There are many other side-effects of phenothiazines, and some of these are also aspects of Parkinsonism. The face may become rigid and emotionless, the voice flat, and there may be difficulty in swallowing saliva, which together with increased production may result in a tendency to dribble. The skin can become greasy as well.

Although it is important never to underestimate the significance of unwanted effects of medicine, it is also important to realize that for most people a balance can be achieved between the desired effects of a drug and its unwanted actions. For now, the use of phenothiazines is the mainstay of the treatment of behavioural disorders and for most people for whom they are prescribed it is possible to arrive at an acceptable compromise.

Another group of medicines that are commonly prescribed for people with dementia are *sleeping pills*. Sometimes the judicious use of a sleeping tablet may prevent a confused person from getting up in the night and causing a disturbance. Nothing is more wearing for a carer than having to cope with very difficult behavioural situations during the day, after having had a disturbed night.

It is important, however, that whatever sleeping medicine is used does not hang over into the next day. Many of the older drugs, including nitrazepam, or Mogadon, which really shouldn't be prescribed for the elderly any longer, have an effect that can hang over into the next day, resulting in sedation and sleepiness during the morning. There are many short-acting night sedatives, such as temazepam, that are less likely to impair a person's intellectual ability the following day, and these are the ones that are best prescribed.

Deciding which dose of which medicine is most appropriate is often a matter of trial and error; those caring for a person with dementia may have to accept that it may take a week or two before the most appropriate dose of night sedation is discovered. It is important that all these medicines are started in the smallest possible dose, usually half that recommended for a young adult; only by slowly increasing from this level can the correct prescription be found.

Most night sedatives have side-effects, one of the most common being a tendency to incontinence. Most elderly people need to get up in the night to go to the bathroom. Drug-induced sleep may lead to the normal arousal mechanisms failing to wake the person concerned when his or her bladder is full, with resulting incontinence. Although most patients with dementia will eventually have this trouble, night sedation can either aggravate it or bring it on earlier. One possible solution is for a spouse or other relative to set an alarm clock for the appropriate time and help the person concerned to use a commode or go to the bathroom. The most appropriate time will vary from person to person and may have to be discovered by trial and error. Unfortunately, waking a person in this way may result in their failing to go back to sleep afterwards, but this is something that can only be tried out. Again, it is important that sleeping tablets are only prescribed for a fixed period and the need for continued prescription considered very carefully.

The Alzheimer's Disease Society has some excellent information and advice sheets that describe in detail the different medicines that may be used to treat behavioural problems, including difficulty with sleep and also the management of depression and anxiety states. Others provide very useful advice about how to manage unusual behaviour and also hallucinations and delusions. This advice will often help avoid the need for drug treatment, or delay the necessity for its prescription.

Support groups

The value of support groups for members of families of patients with dementia is now proved beyond any doubt. As everybody reading this book will be aware, caring for a demented family member creates tremendous practical, psychological and social problems. Carers will talk of a lack of support and information from doctors, poor understanding of the disease processes, depression, feeling trapped, angry and fearful of the sufferer's behavioural problems, the feeling of isolation, and so on. Taking part in a group especially established for the relatives of people with dementia has been shown to be especially beneficial for spouses and others who are the main providers of care. It can reduce their isolation, provide practical and moral support, increase understanding of the disease processes, and help them to become more aware of their own needs.

Although support groups are becoming an increasingly important feature of the care provided by the health service, social services, and voluntary organizations, many relatives will be living in an area where such a group does not exist. If you find yourself in this situation you have three choices. The worst is to do nothing. The most difficult, because of the time required and also because you may well be feeling drained and exhausted, is to start up a group yourself. Or, you can try to persuade somebody else to establish a group. A local social worker, community psychiatric nurse or member of the staff of a day hospital or nursing home may be prepared to act as the focal point for the establishment of a carer's group. It is most likely, however, that you will have to take the initiative yourself, in which case it is a good idea to take advice and counsel from one of the voluntary bodies that already exists to support those caring for relatives with dementia. Probably the most experienced in this field, and certainly the largest in the United Kingdom, is the Alzheimer's Disease Society, whose address and telephone number are included in the list of useful names and addresses at the back of this book. The society has a network of regional offices with trained staff who, although stretched very thinly, will be able to provide information and advice that is relevant to your local area.

A group doesn't have to be large: three or four people, even if they can only meet once or twice a month in one another's houses, may be able to give each other valuable support. The names of others in a similar situation can often be discovered by consultation with your local health visitor, a community psychiatric nurse, the social worker, or by putting up a notice.

Different groups run in different ways, but there are several important points that are common to all those that are most successful. You need to decide realistically how frequently you can meet and how long a meeting should last. Put aside some meetings for general discussion, but try to invite a speaker to at least alternate meetings if possible. Good speakers to have might be the sister of the local psychiatric day hospital, a community psychiatric nurse, an occupational therapist, a doctor, and so on. Each can let you know how he or she works and can give advice on your problems. More importantly you will be able to feed back to them how you feel about what they are doing and very often this will result in a useful rapport. The other advantage of inviting such speakers is that they will inevitably know of many other people who might well be helped by joining your group, and who in turn may help the group.

Although it may be difficult, it is a very good idea to go and talk to people who are running other groups if you can manage this. Even a single visit to an established group in a neighbouring town may give you a lot of useful help.

The first thing to think about, however, is the most difficult problem of all: who will look after those with dementia while their relatives attend the group meetings? In many instances, families or neighbours will be able to help, but there will always be some people who are not in this position and some groups manage to recruit a small body of helpers who are prepared to give up a few hours once a month. These can sometimes be recruited from voluntary organizations such as churches and youth clubs, but it is important to remember the particular qualities that are needed in a person who is going to look after somebody with dementia. If possible, allow them to get to know each other in the presence of the relative who wishes to attend the group, before they are left together for the first time. The best sort of helper in such circumstances is often the relative of a dementia sufferer who has died or moved to institutional care.

Establishing and running a support group can be an extremely rewarding and fulfilling occupation, but it can be very tiring and time-consuming. It may also mean that you will be contacted from time to time by people who have been given your name and who will telephone you for advice about their problems or to inquire about joining the group. Think carefully about this before embarking upon such a course, but do remember that it is usually possible to share out the tasks involved in establishing a group; not only does this relieve the strain on you, but it also adds to the fulfilment experienced by others.

14

Legal and Financial Matters

There are many legal matters that are important, some of which crop up unexpectedly, such as the appropriateness of continuing to drive a car. Wherever possible, however, it is best to try to think ahead and plan before the need arises.

Power of attorney

A full psychological assessment may be necessary before a person with dementia may sign a power of attorney which gives a third party authority to manage the demented person's affairs. This power can be taken out in blanket form, to cover all financial and other important transactions, or may be restricted to specific tasks such as paying regular bills like the gas, electricity and council tax. Inherent in this arrangement is the understanding that the person granting power of attorney to a third party is of sufficiently sound mind to be able to revoke it at any time, and also to be able to control his or her attorney should it be necessary. Anybody who is already significantly intellectually impaired is quite clearly not in a position to protect his or her own interests and under these circumstances it is illegal to enter into such an arrangement.

Similarly, when power of attorney has been granted to a third party by an individual, it ceases to be valid the moment the person on whose behalf it is being exercised becomes unable to manage his or her own affairs through intellectual incapacity. In other words, power of attorney can only remain in force for as long as the person concerned is sound of mind. It is therefore not an appropriate legal instrument to use when a person is already clearly demented. Under these circumstances, it is usually necessary to apply to the Court of Protection.

As many people who grant power of attorney to a relative or other person would have wished their affairs to continue to be administered by their attorney should they become mentally incapacitated, an Act of Parliament came into effect in 1986 allowing a person to grant what is known as an *enduring power of attorney* which continues to be valid whatever the mental ability of the person concerned, but must, however, be drawn up at a time when they are of sound mind.

In many cases therefore it makes sense, before the dementing process is advanced significantly, to establish whether or not the person concerned is sufficiently sound mentally to enable him or her to arrange an enduring power of attorney if the relative or friend is prepared to take on this task. It may save a lot of difficulty later on as the disease progresses, should there be important legal or financial issues that require resolving. The enduring power of attorney will need registering with the Court of Protection when the subject becomes mentally incapable. Your solicitor will advise you about this.

When mental impairment has set in, in the absence of an enduring power of attorneyship it will often be necessary to apply to the Court of Protection on behalf of the person concerned so that the Court can appoint a *receiver* to administer his or her property and affairs. This is usually the next of kin, but need not necessarily be so. There are two advantages to this arrangement. Since the receiver is administering the estate of the person concerned under the direction of the Court, it is unlikely that the receiver will use the person's assets inappropriately. On the other hand the management of a demented person's financial affairs can sometimes cause family dissent and even accusations of impropriety; if all the financial affairs have been scrutinized by the Court, it is very difficult for a third party to make such accusations.

A near relative, intending to make an application for receivership, may approach the Court through a solicitor. Certain forms have to be completed, some by a doctor, but the solicitor will usually arrange this. As with all legal processes, fees are often involved and certainly the solicitor will require payment for his or her part in the application. The Court may also make some charges, but if requested they will be happy to explain these. They produce a series of leaflets as well as a brochure detailing the duties of receivership.

Acting as an agent

When the affairs of a person with dementia are simple and the size of the estate negligible – where restricted, for instance, to the collection of a pension and payment of bills out of it – there is often no need to apply to the Court of Protection. The pension authorities, the Citizens' Advice Bureau, or a well-informed social worker will be able to provide appropriate advice. In general, however, such arrangements are fairly simple to make – for example, the person with dementia, assuming he or she has sufficient intellectual capacity, can inform the local benefits agency of the name of the person who will deal with the finances so that this may be included as an authorization in the order book. The person appointed is then known as the *authorized agent*. It is important to remember, however, that the person on whose behalf this arrangement is being made must have sufficient ability to understand what they are agreeing to. More complicated arrangements may be necessary as the disease progresses but helpful advice can be obtained from the local benefits agency office, the Alzheimer's Disease Society, or a Citizens' Advice Bureau.

Wills

This is something that is best tackled early. As soon as it becomes apparent that a person is beginning to develop a dementia, while they still have some ability to understand the implication of their actions, a solicitor should be consulted if a will needs to be drawn up, or an existing one altered. The situation becomes very complicated if the person with dementia no longer has testamentary capacity, and if he or she does not have a will already, the Court of Protection may have to be approached and they will, in appropriate circumstances, make a statutory will on behalf of the sufferer.

APPENDIX I

Useful Addresses

ALZHEIMER'S DISEASE SOCIETY
The Society, address and
telephone number below,
provides a wealth of information
and advice leaflets for both
relatives and professional carers.
This should be the first point of
contact for anyone wishing for
information on a particular
topic.

Age Concern (*England*)
1268 London Road
London SW16 4ER
Tel: 0181 679 8000

Age Concern Cymru (*Wales*)
4TH Floor, 1 Cathedral Road
Cardiff CF1 9SD
Tel: 01222 371566

Age Concern (*Northern Ireland*)
3 Lower Crescent
Belfast BT7 1NR
Tel: 01232 245729

Age Concern (*Scotland*)
113 Rose Street
Edinburgh EH2 3DT
Tel: 0131 220 3345

**Alzheimer Scotland –
Action on Dementia**
22 Drumsheugh Gardens
Edinburgh EH3 7RN
Tel: 0131 243 1453
Freephone helpline:
0800 317817

Alzheimer's Disease Society
Gordon House
10 Greencoat Place
London SW1P 1PH
Tel: 0171 306 0606

Alzheimer's Disease Society
(*Northern Ireland*)
403 Lisburn Road
Belfast BT9 7EW
Tel: 01232 664100

Alzheimer's Disease Society
(*Wales development office*)
Tonna Hospital
Neath
West Glamorgan SA11 3LX
Tel: 01639 641938

Alzheimer Society of Ireland
Alzheimer House
43 Northumberland Avenue
Dun Laoghaire
Co Dublin, Ireland
Tel: 01 284 6616
From UK: 00 3531 284 6616

**Association of Crossroads
Care Attendants Schemes**
10 Regent Place
Rugby
Warwickshire CV21 2PN
Tel: 01788 573653

Carers Association of Ireland
St Mary's Community Centre
Richmond Hill
Dublin 6
Ireland
Tel: 01 497 4498
From UK: 00 3531 497 4498

Carers National Association
20–25 Glasshouse Yard
London EC1A 4JS
Tel: 0171 490 8818
Helpline: 0171 490 8898

CJD Support Network
Alzheimer's Disease Society
Gordon House
10 Greencoat Place
London SW1P 1PH
Tel: 0171 306 0606

Counsel and Care
Twyman House
16 Bonny Street
London NW1 9PG
Tel: 0171 485 1566

Dementia Relief Trust
Pegasus House
37–43 Sackville Street
London W1X 2DL
Tel: 0171 333 8115

Disabled Living Foundation
380–384 Harrow Road
London W9 2HU
Tel: 0171 289 6111

**The Disablement Income
Group**
5 Archway Business Centre
19–23 Wedmore Street
London N19 4RZ
Tel: 0171 263 3981

DVLA
(Driver and Vehicle Licensing
Agency)
Drivers' Medical Unit
Longview Road
Morriston
Swansea SA99 1TU
Tel: 01792 783686

Help The Aged
St James's Walk
London EC1R 0BE
Tel: 0171 253 0253

MIND
Granta House
15–19 Broadway
Stratford
London E15 4BQ
Tel: 0181 519 2122

Parkinson's Disease Society
22 Upper Woburn Place
London E15 4BQ
Tel: 0171 383 3513

**The Registered Nursing
Homes Association**
Calthorpe House
Hegley Road
Edgbaston
Birmingham B16 8QY
Tel: 0171 263 3981

Stroke Association
Stroke House
Whitecross Street
London EC1Y 8JJ
Tel: 0171 490 7999

**Women's Royal Voluntary
Service**
Milton Hill House
Milton Hill
Abingdon
Oxfordshire OX13 6AF
Tel: 01235 442940

APPENDIX 2

Further Reading

Caring for the person with dementia: a guide for families and other carers, Chris Lay and Bob Woods. Published by Alzheimer's Disease Society in 1994. A 60-page booklet.

Alzheimer's at your fingertips, Harry Cayton, Dr Nori Graham and Dr James Warner. Published by Class Publishing in 1997. A 208-page book arranged in a helpful question and answer format.

Person to person: a guide to the care of those with failing mental powers, Tom Kitwood and Kathleen Bredin. Published by Gale Centre Publications in 1992. A 100-page book.

The 36-hour day: a family guide for caring at home for people with Alzheimer's disease and other confusional illnesses, N. L. Mace, P. V. Rabins, E. McEwen. Published by Age Concern England and Hodder and Stoughton in 1992 (second edition).

It's me Grandma! It's me!, Eileen Evans. Published by Alzheimer's Disease Society in 1992. A 16-page book written in the form of a short story to help children understand the changes that occur with the onset and progression of dementia in a grandparent.

The Long and Winding Road: A Young Person's Guide to Dementia, Jane Gilliard. Published by Wrightson Biomedical Publishing Limited in 1995. A 32-page booklet. This offers suggestions for dealing with the fear and loneliness a young person may experience when dementia strikes a member of their family, or even a friend.

This is just a selection of the ever-increasing literature available for both informal and formal carers. A more extensive list can be obtained from the Alzheimer's Disease Society, who also have what is probably the best professional reading list.

Postscript

The publisher and author hope that you will have found this book helpful, informative and interesting. They would welcome any comments you would like to make that you think might be helpful to others, whether these concern the content or the style. We are sure that there must be room for improvement and it will be our readers, especially those who are carers, who will be able to help us most when we prepare the next edition. We would like to thank the readers who responded to this request in the first edition, without whose help this present edition would be the poorer.

Index